Dr. Tan's Strategy of Twelve Magical Points

ADVANCED PRINCIPLES
AND TECHNIQUES

RICHARD TEH-FU TAN, O.M.D., L.Ac.
Edited by JACKIE W. BENSINGER, L.Ac.

SAN DIEGO, CALIFORNIA

Copyright © 2003 by Richard Tan, O.M.D., L.Ac.

All rights reserved. No part of this book may be used or reproduced, stored in a retrieval system, or transmitted in any form or by any means, electronic, mechanical, photocopying, recording, or otherwise without prior written permission of the publisher.

For information, contact Richard Tan, O.M.D., L.Ac.
4550 Kearny Villa Road, Suite 107, San Diego, CA 92123

Typography: Chuck Surface

Copy Editing: Suzi Surface

Cover Design: Fang-Fang Ting Tan

Printed in San Diego, California

ACKNOWLEDGMENTS

I would like to express my heartfelt thanks to Carrie Denaro for her enthusiasm and skills. Without her generous contribution of time and effort, this project could have never been finalized.

I also want to thank my family and fellow acupuncturists from around the world. Their love, encouragement and support made the publication of this book possible.

Elvis Presley performed the best shows in front of his most inspiring crowds.

Richard Teh-Fu Tan
10-15-2002

Contents

Foreword vii

PART ONE: The Balance Method

About the Balance Method 1

A Brief Introduction to the Five Systems 5

Mirroring Format 19

Imaging Format 23

Four-Segment Timing 31

Yin/Yang Balancing Dynamic 35

Balance Method Treatment Guidelines 41

PART TWO: The Strategy of Twelve Magical Points

The Concept 45

The Mechanics 47

The Patterns 57

Case Studies 71

Appendix A: Pattern Comparison by Sequential Direction of Groups 103

Appendix B: Commonly Asked Questions 107

Foreword

I have compiled information from Chinese medical classics and accumulated more than twenty years experience as an acupuncturist and herbalist. Each of the concepts I have taught have been "meridian-driven" and designed to achieve high clinical efficacy. These include the I-Ching/Ba Gua, Five Systems, Imaging and Mirroring Formats, Yin/Yang Balancing Dynamic and Four-Segment Timing.

However, in the past few years more and more patients have come into my office with modern, idiopathic illnesses such as chronic fatigue syndrome, fibromyalgia and autoimmune disorders. These patients often present with symptoms that make it difficult to pinpoint the meridian responsible for the imbalance. Even the pulse and tongue do not reveal a clear TCM diagnosis or suggest a specific complication. In these cases, it is no longer a clear choice of treating pain versus internal pathology.

Typically, an acupuncturist diagnoses an imbalance according to *which* channel is affected. Often pain is the body's way of leading us to the most direct road that heals the root imbalance.

Remember, the basic acupuncture text states the ben (root) can also be treated by addressing the biao (branch.) Therefore, treatments that regulate affected meridians also serve to correct underlying imbalances. Unfortunately, this determination of a treatment strategy can be perplexing if the patient is not experiencing pain, or if the pain is all over the body.

As more of these cases entered my clinic, I asked myself a few simple questions: Why not develop a system that can balance the entire body in the same treatment? Why not choose points from each of the 12 meridians? Why not increase the healing capacity by applying concepts that already proved to be clinically effective? I developed the Strategy of Twelve Magical Points to answer these questions. It utilizes all the meridians and is based on the Four-Segment Timing (seasons and time of day), Imaging and Mirroring Formats and the Yin/Yang Balancing Dynamic.

Prior to revealing my invention, I have practiced this method on hundreds of patients with astonishing results. In sharing this strategy, it is my hope that many more patients and practitioners will experience widespread benefits. My dream is that more acupuncturists will become inspired to create their own treatment strategies with equally amazing clinical outcomes. As a Chinese proverb says: I am tossing out one piece of brick with the hopes of motivating other practitioners to contribute beautiful pieces of jade. Together, the treasure of acupuncture prosperity will be built.

Richard Teh-Fu Tan, O.M.D., L.Ac.

Editor's Note

Dr. Richard Teh-Fu Tan has taught the basic Five Systems of the Balance Method to thousands of people for the past ten years. I had the great fortune to attend hundreds of these classes during my seven years as his apprentice. I was always amazed at Dr. Tan's ability to continually fine-tune his teachings to enhance the audience's understanding of his method. It seemed as if this master acupuncturist would try anything from laughter to tears to inspire us to see the myriad of choices available for treating patients outside the realm of our basic training.

In each of the Five Systems we see how Chinese Medicine uncovers the healing connections and meridian networks already provided by nature. Dr. Tan's acupuncture method, Chi Cultivation format and life philosophy all stem from one basic premise: Under the right conditions, the internal healing system naturally adjusts imbalances in the body with little interference from the outside. I believe that finding the combinations of variables to create this natural order motivated Dr. Tan to develop this extraordinary new system of the Balance Method.

Using the Strategy of Twelve Magical Points, he teaches us how to build treatments for complex conditions that clinically confound most of us. Dr. Tan has ingeniously devised 16 sets of treatments based on the Tai Ji that include all 12 meridians and utilize the Five Transporting points. His method addresses the concepts of time and space and prepares a dynamic framework to furnish kinetic energy for altering the human condition.

This book is the product of years of study and research by Dr. Richard Teh-Fu Tan, a Grand Master of acupuncture. As a result of his dedication and innovative treatments, we can now confidently face our patients suffering from unbearable pain and complex internal disorders

Jackie W. Bensinger, L.Ac.

How to Use This Book

Dr. Tan's Strategy of Twelve Magical Points is designed for acupuncturists who may or may not be familiar with the Balance Method; however, an elementary working knowledge of the basic Balance Method is essential in order to understand the strategy. Part One of this text introduces the basics of the Balance Method: the Five Systems, the Mirroring and Imaging Formats, the Yin/Yang Balancing Dynamic and Four-Segment Timing. Before delving into the Strategy of Twelve Magical Points, we suggest reading these sections and applying this method to your practice.

Part Two of the text is devoted to the theory and explanation behind the Strategy of the Twelve Magical Points, including diagrams of the eight patterns that make up the system. Twenty-four case studies are included to illustrate the technique and facilitate understanding of pattern selection.

Additional Support

Reference material on the Balance Method can be found online at www.drtanshow.com. An online forum is also available on the site to connect practitioners who want to ask questions or share cases. Dr. Tan's two previous texts, *Twelve and Twelve in Acupuncture* and *Twenty-Four More in Acupuncture,* are great references for effective points used in everyday practice. Students of the Balance Method can also use these texts as study tools for understanding the theory behind the points discussed in these books.

Reading this book is sufficient to apply the Five Systems of the Balance Method and the Twelve Points Magical Strategy. However, classes on the Balance Method are recommended for practitioners who wish to obtain a more in-depth study of the systems and underlying theory. From one viewpoint, the method merely involves following simple concepts and utilizing logical systems. However, students who choose to look from a broader perspective will discover that it contains a multi-dimensional quality. Learning this new strategy to a degree beyond simple recognition ensures superior clinical efficacy and encourages further research.

PART ONE:
The Balance Method

About the Balance Method 1

A Brief Introduction to the Five Systems 5

Mirroring Format 19

Imaging Format 23

Four-Segment Timing 31

Yin/Yang Balancing Dynamic 35

Balance Method Treatment Guidelines 41

About the Balance Method

The Balance Method is a series of acupuncture systems rooted in the concept of healing the body by balancing meridians. This revolutionary approach contains logical steps for constructing an acupuncture treatment in an easy-to-use format. The basis of the Balance Method relies on a simple two-step process. First, the Five Systems are used to determine which meridian(s) should be needled. These systems form the basic structure of your acupuncture treatment. Then, the Mirroring and Imaging Formats assist in point selections along those chosen meridians.

Dr. Richard Teh-Fu Tan is the first person to assemble this body of information into a systematic method and translate it into the English language. Classical Chinese texts make reference to the concepts that form the basis of the Five Systems of the Balance Method; however, the information is scattered and has never been compiled into a practical treatment format. For example, the Biao-Li (Interior/Exterior concept) is taught in basic acupuncture texts, but the correct usage is never mentioned. Dr. Tan studied, researched and applied these concepts for more than 20 years. His correlations and organization of the material comprise the core of the Balance Method.

Dr. Tan also has developed several Advanced Systems to balance internal disorders by various means of trigram calculation. For example, the six yaos of each hexagram may be modified to represent particular meridians. These relationships are then applied to balance the body according to the Five Systems or the seasons. The Strategy of Twelve Magical Points is Dr. Tan's most recent addition to the Balance Method. It is the absolute culmination of his career as a doctor and systems engineer. No other treatment strategy exists which integrates all twelve meridians, the element of time, and the Mirroring and Imaging Formats. The result of this creation is an immediate shift in the body, correcting numerous and complex imbalances.

Distal points are used exclusively in all systems of the Balance Method. This means that external and internal disorders are treated effectively without using even one local point. The Five Systems, or any of the advanced systems, provide relationships to affected meridian(s) and balance disorders using a see-saw effect. In the ancient medical text, the *Nei Jing,* the limb is regarded as the root and the trunk as the branch. This concept is the foundation for treatment of the whole body with the use of distal points.

Among the many types of pain treated successfully by the Balance Method are migraine headaches, fibromyalgia, sciatica, arthritis, musculoskeletal pain and phantom-limb pain. Pain-like sensations such as numbness, tingling, burning, aching, itching and cramping are also effectively treated by balancing the affected meridian.

Furthermore, internal conditions such as nausea, asthma, edema, irritable bowel syndrome, insomnia, palpitations, sore

About the Balance Method

throat, cough, diarrhea, menorrhagia, P.M.S., menopause, prostatitis and impotence can be treated. Skin conditions including acne, rashes, boils, bumps, pustules, flaking, and swelling also respond well to Balance Method treatments. In short, the Balance Method addresses any condition that is relieved by acupuncture.

Correct diagnosis is crucial for any doctor. For an acupuncturist, determination of the sick meridian is the first step to providing fast relief for the patient's suffering. ***The term "sick meridian" refers to the affected channel.*** Imbalances can manifest along a sick meridian as pain, swelling or rashes. For example, if a rash covers the area of LI4 to SJ4, then LI and SJ are the sick meridians.

If the patient has an internal pathology without the presence of pain, the basic Five Element approach to pulse taking is very helpful. The channel related to the specific pulse quality will assist in determining the sick meridian. In addition, the basic diagnostic methods are essential: asking, listening, observing and palpating.

Wiry	Liver and Gall Bladder channels
Bouncy	Heart and Small Intestine channels
Thready	Spleen and Stomach channels
Floating	Lung and Large Intestine channels
Deep	Kidney and Urinary Bladder channels

Basic Five Element Pulses

Once the sick meridian(s) have been determined, the Five Systems are used to analyze the choices of meridians to treat. The next section, *A Brief Introduction to the Five Systems,* discusses the various meridian relationships and the approach to determine the meridian(s) to needle. The following sections,

Dr. Tan's Strategy of Twelve Magical Points

Mirroring Format, Imaging Format and *Four-Segment Timing,* will cover point selection. The *Yin/Yang Balancing Dynamic* places the selected points in a specific arrangement designed to create an energetic attraction that balances the body. The *Balance Method Treatment Guidelines* is found at the end of these sections and provides a step-by-step summary to formulate your treatment strategy.

The Balance Method results in a rapid shift of the body into a state of equilibrium. Initial follow-up treatments are required two to three times per week to maintain this condition. The total number of treatments necessary depends on the imbalance and the individual response of the patient. Most imbalances are relieved within ten to twelve treatments over a period of one month. Generally, patients who do not respond within eight treatments may not benefit from acupuncture. A small percentage of patients have a "reaction" to the Balance Method. This means their condition may worsen for 24-48 hours and then improve. Some patients notice no change for 24-48 hours and then later improve.

A Brief Introduction to the Five Systems

The Five Systems of the Balance Method provide the meridian connections that are used to systematically choose which channel(s) should be treated. The Five Systems achieve a dynamic balance by pairing a sick meridian with various balancing meridians that are pre-arranged in each particular system. These five relationships among the twelve channels include attributes of the meridian such as organ specification, yin or yang quality, anatomical location, Chinese clock positions, and hand or foot association. The Chinese meridian names are essential to distinguish channel relationship in the Balance Method: Tai Yin, Jue Yin, Shao Yin, Yang Ming, Shao Yang and Tai Yang.

System 1 pairs channels sharing the same meridian name, such as Hand and Foot Tai Yin. System 2 pairs opposite channels according to the Chinese meridian names, such as Hand Tai Yin with Foot Tai Yang. System 3 pairs organs that share the familiar Zang Fu relationships, such as Hand Tai Yin (Lung) with Hand Yang Ming (Large Intestine). System 4 pairs opposite meridians on the Chinese clock, such as Foot Tai Yin with Hand Shao Yang. Lastly, System 5 pairs neighbors on the

Dr. Tan's Strategy of Twelve Magical Points

Chinese Clock, such as Foot Tai Yin with Hand Shao Yin. Balance is achieved by combining the affected meridian with the appropriate channels according to the specifications of each system.

Precise determination of the sick meridian is vital to achieve successful results using the Balance Method. Ask the patient to pinpoint or trace the problem area with one finger in order to locate the specific channel(s) affected. For example, a sprained wrist could involve one or more of six meridians: Hand Tai Yin, Hand Jue Yin, Hand Shao Yin, Hand Yang Ming, Hand Shao Yang, and Hand Tai Yang. When the affected area is between channels, the treatment of choice would be between the balancing channels. For example, in System 1, wrist pain between Hand Yang Ming and Hand Shao Yang can be treated at an ashi area on the opposite ankle between Foot Yang Ming and Foot Shao Yang.

Each system contains a well-organized format to determine channel relationships; Systems 1, 2 and 3 are based on I-Ching theory, while the Chinese clock is the framework for Systems 4 and 5. In this text, the presence of the Five Systems facilitates understanding for the use of the Twelve Points Strategy.

A Brief Introduction to the Five Systems

System 1: Chinese Meridian Name-Sharing

In System 1 the sick meridian and the needled meridian have the same Chinese meridian name, excluding Du and Ren. A hand channel balances a foot channel and vice versa. Yin channels balance yin channels and yang channels balance yang channels.

For example, a problem in the Hand Tai Yin channel (Lung) is balanced by the Foot Tai Yin (Spleen) channel. Any two channels with the same Chinese meridian name balance each other.

Needle: Opposite side

Sick Meridian	Needled Meridian
Du	Ren
Ren	Du
Hand Tai Yin/Lung	Foot Tai Yin/Spleen
Foot Tai Yin/Spleen	Hand Tai Yin/Lung
Foot Yang Ming/Stomach	Hand Yang Ming/Large Intestine
Hand Yang Ming/Large Intestine	Foot Yang Ming/Stomach
Hand Shao Yin/Heart	Foot Shao Yin/Kidney
Foot Shao Yin/Kidney	Hand Shao Yin/Heart
Hand Tai Yang/Small Intestine	Foot Tai Yang/Urinary Bladder
Foot Tai Yang/Urinary Bladder	Hand Tai Yang/Small Intestine
Hand Jue Yin/Pericardium	Foot Jue Yin/Liver
Foot Jue Yin/Liver	Hand Jue Yin/Pericardium
Hand Shao Yang/San Jiao	Foot Shao Yang/Gall Bladder
Foot Shao Yang/Gall Bladder	Hand Shao Yang/San Jiao

System 1—Chinese Meridian Name-Sharing

Dr. Tan's Strategy of Twelve Magical Points

Example for System 1

A patient presents with left-sided tennis elbow on Hand Yang Ming (Large Intestine) in the area of LI 11. The needled meridian is Foot Yang Ming (Stomach) on the right side. Point selection is accomplished by using the Mirroring Format, as discussed in a later section. ST35, or an ashi point near ST35, would be the appropriate knee point to treat the elbow pain.

A Brief Introduction to the Five Systems

System 2: Bie-Jing/Branching Channels

System 2 illustrates the mutual attraction of Tai Yin with Tai Yang, Jue Yin with Yang Ming, and Shao Yin with Shao Yang.

Hand channels are paired with foot channels and foot channels are paired with hand channels. For example, Hand Shao Yang links with Foot Shao Yin. In this system, yin channels balance yang channels and yang channels balance yin channels.

Needle: Either side

Sick Meridian	Needled Meridian
Hand Tai Yin/Lung	Foot Tai Yang/Urinary Bladder
Foot Tai Yang/Urinary Bladder	Hand Tai Yin/Lung
Hand Tai Yang/Small Intestine	Foot Tai Yin/Spleen
Foot Tai Yin/Spleen	Hand Tai Yang/Small Intestine
Hand Shao Yin/Heart	Foot Shao Yang/Gall Bladder
Foot Shao Yang/Gall Bladder	Hand Shao Yin/Heart
Hand Shao Yang/San Jiao	Foot Shao Yin/Kidney
Foot Shao Yin/Kidney	Hand Shao Yang/San Jiao
Hand Jue Yin/Pericardium	Foot Yang Ming/Stomach
Foot Yang Ming/Stomach	Hand Jue Yin/Pericardium
Foot Jue Yin/Liver	Hand Yang Ming/Large Intestine
Hand Yang Ming/Large Intestine	Foot Jue Yin/Liver

System 2—Bie-Jing/Branching Channels

Example for System 2

A patient presents with a sprained ankle on Foot Shao Yang at GB40 on the right side. The needled meridian is the Hand Shao Yin. The appropriate point to use is HT7 on the right or left side. Needle the side that is more ashi.

System 3: Biao-Li or Interior/Exterior Pairs

System 3 represents the interior/exterior pairs that are easily recognized as the Zang Fu organ relationships. The needled meridian is the Biao-Li counterpart to the sick meridian. For example, Liver treats Gall Bladder and Gall Bladder treats Liver. Yin channels balance yang channels and yang channels balance yin channels.

This is the only one of the Five Systems in which hand channels pair with hand channels and foot channels pair with foot channels. For example, Lung treats Large Intestine and Large Intestine treats Lung. Though the Biao-Li concept is familiar, needling the opposite side from the affected channel is not common knowledge.

Needle: Opposite side

Sick Meridian	Needled Meridian
Hand Tai Yin/Lung	Hand Yang Ming/Large Intestine
Hand Yang Ming/Large Intestine	Hand Tai Yin/Lung
Hand Shao Yin/Heart	Hand Tai Yang/Small Intestine
Hand Tai Yang/Small Intestine	Hand Shao Yin/Heart
Hand Jue Yin/Percardium	Hand Shao Yang/San Jiao
Hand Shao Yang/San Jiao	Hand Jue Yin/Percardium
Foot Tai Yin/Spleen	Foot Yang Ming/Stomach
Foot Yang Ming/Stomach	Foot Tai Yin/Spleen
Foot Shao Yin/Kidney	Foot Tai Yang/Urinary Bladder
Foot Tai Yang/Urinary Bladder	Foot Shao Yin/Kidney
Foot Jue Yin/Liver	Foot Shao Yang/Gall Bladder
Foot Shao Yang/Gall Bladder	Foot Jue Yin/Liver

System 3—Biao-Li or Interior/Exterior

Example for System 3

A patient presents with left-sided knee pain on the Foot Jue Yin channel at LV8. The needled meridian is Foot Shao Yang on the right side. The appropriate point is GB34 using the Mirroring format.

Dr. Tan's Strategy of Twelve Magical Points

System 4: Chinese Clock Opposites

System 4 uses the format of the Chinese Clock to locate the needled channel. The sick meridian on one side of the clock pairs with the needled meridian on the opposite side. Traditionally, the flow of chi creates a twelve hour difference between the clock pairs. For example, Liver time is between the hours of 1:00-3:00am. and Small Intestine time is from 1:00-3:00pm. Therefore, Foot Jue yin balances Hand Tai yang and vice versa. The pairs are opposite each other on the Chinese Clock. ***The actual time of the acupuncture treatment is not considered in applying this system of the Balance Method. The treatment is effective at any time.***

Yin meridians balance yang meridians and yang meridians balance yin meridians. Hand channels are paired with foot channels and foot channels are paired with hand channels. Several pairs within the Chinese Clock Opposites format overlap with System 2 (Bie-Jing, Branching Channels).

A Brief Introduction to the Five Systems

Needle: Either side

Sick Meridian	Needled Meridian
*Hand Tai Yin/Lung	Foot Tai Yang/Urinary Bladder
Hand Yang Ming/Large Intestine	Foot Shao Yin/Kidney
*Foot Yang Ming/Stomach	Hand Jue Yin/Pericardium
Foot Tai Yin/Spleen	Hand Shao Yang/San Jiao
*Hand Shao Yin/Heart	Foot Shao Yang/Gall Bladder
Hand Tai Yang/Small Intestine	Foot Jue Yin/Liver
*Foot Tai Yang/Urinary Bladder	Hand Tai Yin/Lung
Foot Shao Yin/Kidney	Hand Yang Ming/Large Intestine
*Hand Jue Yin/Percardium	Foot Yang Ming/Stomach
Hand Shao Yang/San Jiao	Foot Tai Yin/Spleen
*Foot Shao Yang/Gall Bladder	Hand Shao Yin/Heart
Foot Jue Yin/Liver	Hand Tai Yang/Small Intestine

System 4—Chinese Clock Opposites

*These meridian pairs share the same relationship as the meridian pairs in System 2 (Bie-Jing/Branching Channels).

Dr. Tan's Strategy of Twelve Magical Points

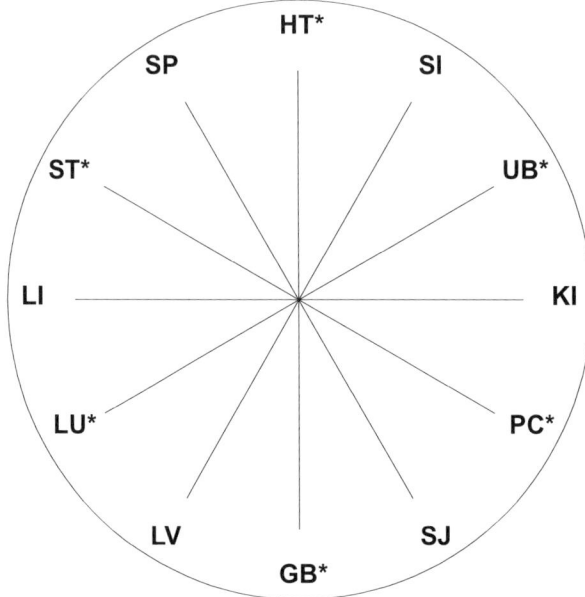

Chinese Clock Opposites

*These meridian pairs share the same relationship as the meridian pairs in System 2 (Bie-Jing/Branching Channels).

Example for System 4

A patient presents with pain along the Hand Tai Yang/Small Intestine channel at SI12-SI14 on the left scapula. The needled meridian is Foot Jue Yin/Liver channel on the left side or the right side. Using the Imaging Format, the appropriate point is around LV4-LV5.

A Brief Introduction to the Five Systems

System 5: Chinese Clock Neighbors

System 5 uses the arrangement of the neighbor system on the Chinese Clock. Hand channels are paired with foot channels and foot channels are paired with hand channels. Yin channels balance yin channels and yang channels balance yang channels. For example, Hand Tai Yin treats Foot Jue Yin and vice versa. Several Chinese Clock Neighbors overlap with System 1 (Chinese Meridian Name-Sharing).

The actual time of the acupuncture treatment is not considered in applying this system of the Balance Method. The treatment is effective at any time.

Needle: Opposite side

Sick Meridian	Needled Meridian
Hand Tai Yin/Lung	Foot Jue Yin/Liver
*Hand Yang Ming/Large Intestine	Foot Yang Ming/Stomach
*Foot Yang Ming/Stomach	Hand Yang Ming/Large Intestine
Foot Tai Yin/Spleen	Hand Shao Yin/Heart
Hand Shao Yin/Heart	Foot Tai Yin/Spleen
*Hand Tai Yang/Small Intestine	Foot Tai Yang/Urinary Bladder
*Foot Tai Yang/Urinary Bladder	Hand Tai Yang/Small Intestine
Foot Shao Yin/Kidney	Hand Jue Yin/Pericardium
Hand Jue Yin/Pericardium	Foot Shao Yin/Kidney
*Hand Shao Yang/San Jiao	Foot Shao Yang/Gall Bladder
*Foot Shao Yang/Gall Bladder	Hand Shao Yang/San Jiao
Foot Jue Yin/Liver	Hand Tai Yin/Lung

System 5—Chinese Clock Neighbors

*These meridian pairs share the same relationship as the meridian pairs in System 1 (Chinese Meridian Name Sharing).

Dr. Tan's Strategy of Twelve Magical Points

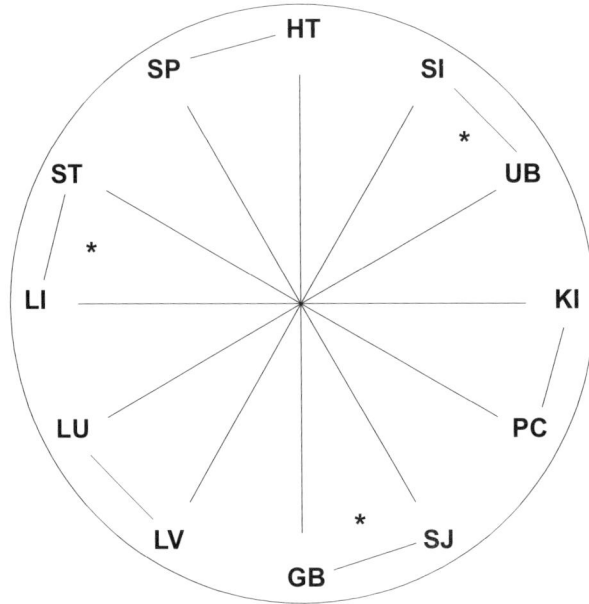

Chinese Clock Neighbors

*These meridian pairs share the same relationship as the meridian pairs in System 1 (Chinese Meridian Name Sharing).

Example for System 5

Patient presents with hepatitis on the Foot Jue Yin/Liver channel. The needled meridian is Hand Tai Yin, the Lung meridian. The appropriate point to needle is LU6 using the Imaging Format.

A Brief Introduction to the Five Systems

Summary of the Five Systems of the Balance Method

System Name	System Features
System 1 Chinese Meridian Name-Sharing	Pairs channels with same Chinese meridian name. Hand channels treat foot channels and vice versa. Yin channels treat yin channels, and yang treat yang. Treats contralateral side.
System 2 Bie-Jing / Branching Meridians	Pairs channels with specific Chinese meridian relationships. Hand channels treat foot channels and vice versa. Yin channels treat yang channels, and yang treat yin. Treats ipsilateral or contralateral side.
System 3 Biao-Li or Interior/Exterior pairs	Pairs channels with Zang Fu organ relationships. Hand channels treat hand channels, and foot treat foot. Yin channels treat yang channels, and yang treat yin. Treats contralateral side.
System 4 Chinese Clock Opposites	Pairs channels on opposite sides of the Chinese clock. Hand channels treat foot channels and vice versa. Yin channels treat yang channels, and yang treat yin. Treats ipsilateral or contralateral side.
System 5 Chinese Clock Neighbors	Pairs neighbors on the Chinese clock. Hand channels treat foot channels and vice versa. Yin channels treat yin channels, and yang treat yang. Treats contralateral side.

Dr. Tan's Strategy of Twelve Magical Points

MIRRORING FORMAT

The Five Systems provide five different approaches to determine which meridian(s) should be needled. The Mirroring Format is designed to specify the area of the limb that will respond positively and balance the problem. The mirroring concept is derived from the body's remarkable ability to reflect tenderness, weakness or tightness in an area on a limb distal from the sick meridian.

To use the Mirroring Format, first match the sick meridian to an appropriate needled meridian by application of one the Five Systems. Then mirror the "sick" area to a corresponding anatomical location on the chosen needled meridian. Exact point selection is determined in many cases by checking for "ashi" points in the mirrored area rather than the standard acupuncture points.

In most cases, the Mirroring Format balances the upper limb to the lower limb or the lower limb to the upper limb. System 3 is the only exception that balances upper limb to upper limb and lower limb to lower limb.

Dr. Tan's Strategy of Twelve Magical Points

The term "limb" includes all parts of the limb such as the fingers, toes, wrists, ankles, elbows, knees, shoulders and hips. For example, if the injured area is the knee, the opposite limb is the elbow. Refer to the Summary of the Five Systems to determine which systems use ipsilateral or contralateral sides. To apply the Reverse Mirroring Format, invert the mirrored limb to be needled. For example, a foot problem can be treated by reversing the upper limb and needling the shoulder.

Mirroring Format		
Finger	↔	Toe
Hand	↔	Foot
Wrist	↔	Ankle
Forearm	↔	Lower Leg
Elbow	↔	Knee
Upper Arm	↔	Thigh
Shoulder	↔	Hip

Reverse Mirroring Format		
Finger	↔	Top of Hip
Hand	↔	Hip
Wrist	↔	Hip Joint
Forearm	↔	Thigh
Elbow	↔	Knee
Upper Arm	↔	Lower Leg
Shoulder	↔	Ankle

Mirroring Format

Case Studies Using the Five Systems and the Mirroring Format

Example: Right-sided ankle pain on the foot Shao Yang/Gall Bladder meridian.

Affected area	System 1	System 2	System 3	System 4	System 5
GB40 (R)	SJ4 (L)	HT7 (R or L)	LV4 (L)	HT7 (R or L)	SJ4 (L)

Example: Left-sided knee pain on the foot Shao Yin/Kidney meridian.

Affected area	System 1	System 2	System 3	System 4	System 5
KI10 (L)	HT3 (R)	SJ10 (L or R)	UB40 (R)	LI11 (L or R)	PC3 (R)

Example: Right-sided shoulder pain on the hand Yang Ming meridian.

Affected area	System 1	System 2	System 3	System 4	System 5
LI15 (R)	ST31 (L)	LV10/11 (L or R)	LU2 (L)	KI 11A* (L or R)	ST31 (L)

*A = Ashi point in the region of the standard point location

Example: Right-sided shoulder pain on the hand Yang Ming meridian. *Reverse Mirroring Format.*

Affected area	System 1	System 2	System 3	System 4	System 5
LI15 (R)	ST41 (L)	LV4 (L or R)	LU 9 (L)	KI3 (L or R)	ST41 (L)

Dr. Tan's Strategy of Twelve Magical Points

IMAGING FORMAT

The Imaging Format is a method of point selection which images the sick area of the body onto a different area of the body. The corresponding area on the needled meridian often reflects tenderness, weakness or tightness from the affected meridian of the head, trunk or limb.

Unlike the Mirroring Format, the Imaging Format is not restricted to balancing limb with limb. The head can balance the limb and the limb can balance the head; the trunk can balance the limb and the limb can balance the trunk.

To use the Imaging Format, first match the sick meridian to a needled meridian using the Five Systems. Then imagine the "sick" area superimposed on the head, the trunk or a limb. For example, if the sick area is on the face, place the image of the face on the leg or the arm. If the head is superimposed on the whole leg, then eye level is located at the knee. Exact point selection is determined in many cases by checking for ashi points on the appropriate meridians rather than the standard acupuncture points.

Dr. Tan's Strategy of Twelve Magical Points

Reverse Imaging Format can be applied by inverting images. For example, when overlaying the image of the torso onto the upper limb, the genitals are level with the wrist and the neck is level with the shoulder. Therefore, genital pain can be treated by needling the wrist. If the images are reversed, the genitals are now level with the shoulder and the neck is level with the wrist. Therefore, the genital pain can also be treated by needling the shoulder.

Rotation and inversion of the image of the trunk allows the lower abdomen to be treated by needling the upper back. To begin, overlay an image of the front of the torso onto the back of the body. The lower abdomen would appear level with the lumbar vertebrae in this image. Then invert the torso so that the clavicles are level with the buttocks and the low abdomen is level with the scapula and shoulders. In this way, the lower half of the anterior trunk of the body is treated by the upper half of the posterior trunk, and vice versa.

Generally, if your chosen image is an inconvenient location for needling and requires the removal of clothes, then an image that is more easily accessible can be selected. If three or more treatments have not produced any response from the patient, select another image or reverse and/or rotate the current image. With a few needles the whole body can be treated with a multitude of combinations using the Imaging Format.

Imaging Format

Image of Upper Limb to Head and Trunk

Needled Area	Sick Area	
	Image	Reverse Image
Finger	Testicles and anus	Top of head
Hand	Genitals, coccyx, sacrum	Head and base of skull
Wrist	Bladder area, lumbo-sacral area	Neck and neck joint
Forearm	Lower abdomen, lower back	Upper abdomen, rib cage, chest, mid-upper back
Elbow	Umbilicus level, Lumbar 2, waist	Umbilicus level, Lumbar 2, waist
Upper arm	Upper abdomen, rib cage, chest, mid-upper back	Lower abdomen, lower back
Shoulder	Neck, jaw, base of skull	Sacrum, genitals, coccyx
Top of shoulder	Top of head	Testicles and anus

Image of Lower Limb to Head and Trunk

Needled Area	Sick Area	
	Image	Reverse Image
Toe	Testicles and anus	Top of head
Foot	Genitals, coccyx, sacrum	Head and base of skull
Ankle	Bladder area, lumbo-sacral area	Neck and neck joint
Lower Leg	Lower abdomen, lower back	Upper abdomen, rib cage, chest, mid-upper back
Knee	Umbilicus level, Lumbar 2, waist	Umbilicus level, Lumbar 2, waist
Upper leg	Upper abdomen, rib cage, chest, mid-upper back	Lower abdomen, lower back
Hip joint	Neck, jaw, base of skull	Sacrum, genitals, coccyx
Top of hip	Top of head	Testicles and anus

Imaging Format

Image of Head to Upper and Lower Limbs

Needled Area	Sick Area	
	Lower Limb	Upper Limb
Top of Head/Du20	Hip	Shoulder
Forehead Level	Thigh	Upper arm
Eye, Ear, Occiput	Knee	Elbow
Nose Level	Lower leg (upper portion)	Forearm (upper portion)
Mouth Level	Lower leg (lower portion)	Forearm (lower portion)
Chin Level	Ankle	Wrist

Reverse Image of Head to Upper and Lower Limbs

Needled Area	Sick Area	
	Lower Limb	Upper Limb
Top of Head/Du20	Ankle	Wrist
Forehead Level	Lower leg	Forearm
Eye, Ear, Occiput	Knee	Elbow
Nose Level	Thigh (lower portion)	Upper arm (lower portion)
Mouth Level	Thigh (upper portion)	Upper arm (upper portion)
Chin Level	Hip	Shoulder

Case Studies Using the Five Systems and the Imaging Formats

Example: Shingle pain on the rib cage at LV14

	System 1	System 2	System 3	System 4	System 5
Image:	PC3A↑	LI 13A	GB33A	SI8A↑	LU5A↑
Reverse image:	PC3A↓	LI7A	GB34A	SI7A	LU5A↓

Example: Headache at GB8

	System 1	System 2	System 3	System 4	System 5
Image:	SJ 10A	HT3A	LV8A	HT3A	SJ10A

Example: Neck pain on UB channel, C5 level.

	System 1	System 2	System 3	System 4	System 5
Image:	SI9-10A	LU1-2A	KI10-11A (Top of upper leg)	LU1-2A	SI9-10A
Reverse image:	SI5-6A	LU8A	KI3-7A	LU8A	SI5-6A

*A = Ashi point in the region of the standard point location
*↑ ↓ = Ashi point located above or below area of standard point location

Dr. Tan's Strategy of Twelve Magical Points

FOUR-SEGMENT TIMING

Four-Segment Timing is the third method that assists in point selection. It is based on the relationship between the rhythms of Nature and the Five Shu-Transporting points. Man is connected to the cycles of the Universe by his biology. Though not fully understood, human sensitivity to changes in the Earth's magnetism from solar and lunar activity has been shown in studies for over fifty years. Sleep cycles, hormone levels and mental states are among the many human conditions affected by changes in the Earth's magnetic and electrical fields.

In Chinese philosophy, the Tai Ji symbol illustrates the foundation for these natural cycles and reveals relationships between the 24-hour day and the four seasons. The greatest yang, expansiveness or brightness, is summer or noontime; the greatest yin, contraction or darkness, is winter or midnight.

Dr. Tan's Strategy of Twelve Magical Points

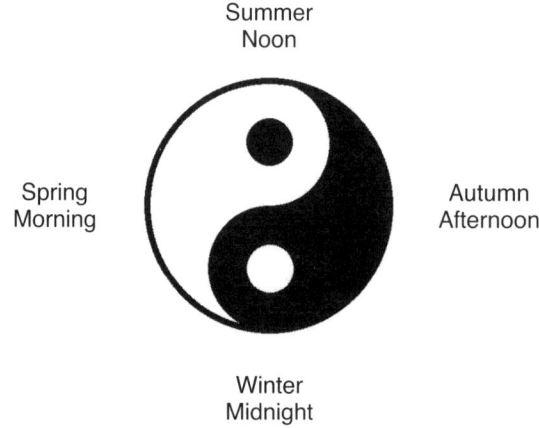

Tai Ji Symbol and Cyclical Relationships

Since the second century, acupuncture systems have addressed the body's responsiveness to these cyclical rhythms of the days and seasons. Four-Segment Timing first appeared in references from the *Nan Jing* relating the use of the Five Shu-Transporting points to the four phases of the day/night cycle and the four seasons.

As illustrated in the following chart, two groups of Shu points share each segment of the four phases. In the Four-Segment Timing, Jing-Well and Ying-Spring points are used during the late night, midnight and winter. Ying-Spring and Shu-Stream points are applied in the early morning and spring. The Shu-Stream and Jing-River points are used in the late morning, early afternoon and summer. The Jing-River and He-Sea points are utilized in the late afternoon, evening or autumn.

Four-Segment Timing

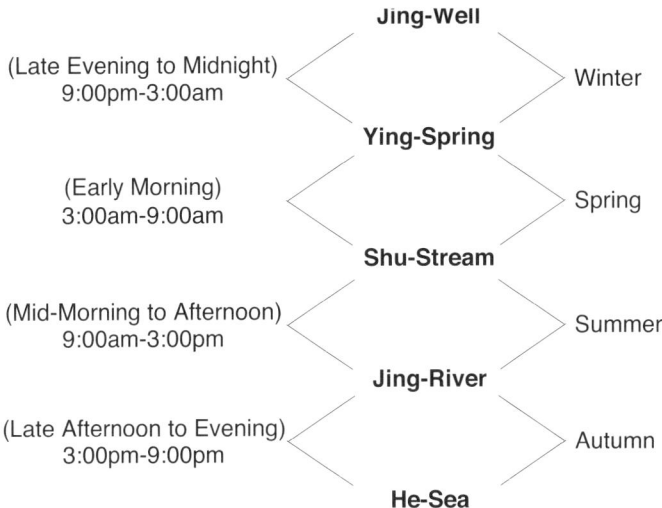

Relationship of Five Shu Points and Four-Segment Timing

An entire meridian can be treated and balanced by use of the points based on Four-Segment Timing. Points from these four groups can be used alone or in combination with other points to influence the whole meridian. Disorders caused or exacerbated by seasonal changes such as allergies, joint pain, muscle aches and certain types of depression are especially relieved by treatment application according to the concept of Four-Segment Timing.

Two of the Five Systems within the Balance Method also address meridian selection based on natural timing by using the Chinese Clock. In an Advanced System of the Balance Method, the Seasonal Balancing System, the hexagram of the current season is used to balance the hexagram of the affected meridian.

Dr. Tan's Strategy of Twelve Magical Points

Case Study Using the Five Systems and the Four-Segment Format

Example: Migraine headache located on the Foot Shao Yang meridian.

	System 1	System 2	System 3	System 4	System 5
Midnight/Winter Jing-Well or Ying-Spring	SJ1 or SJ2	HT9 or HT8	LV1 or LV2	HT9 or HT8	SJ1 or SJ2
Morning/Spring Ying-Spring or Shu-Stream	SJ2 or SJ3	HT8 or HT7	LV2 or LV3	HT8 or HT7	SJ2 or SJ3
Noon/Summer Shu-Stream or Jing-River	SJ3 or SJ6	HT7 or HT4	LV3 or LV4	HT7 or HT4	SJ3 or SJ6
Evening/Fall Jing River or He-Sea	SJ6 or SJ10	HT4 or HT3	LV4 or LV8	HT4 or HT3	SJ6 or SJ10

Yin/Yang Balancing Dynamic

As explained in the preceding sections, the needled meridian(s) are determined using the Five Systems. Then, specific points are selected using the Mirroring Format, Imaging Format or Four-Segment Timing. As a final step, the chosen points are then placed on a diagram called the Yin/Yang Balancing Dynamic. This format engages the two fundamental energies of yin and yang, assists with meridian selection in terms of the layout, and launches the treatment strategy into motion.

In order to understand the application of yin and yang in the Balance Method, it is important to look at the history of these concepts. The Tai Ji symbol originates from the wisdom of the *I-Ching* and represents the ebb and flow of the yin/yang forces. The Tai Ji forms the foundation of Chinese Medicine. It illustrates the concept of mutual attraction of opposites and dynamic balance. The shifting balance of the Tai Ji holds the metaphor for life processes. This can be found in our relationships, the internal cycles of the body, the seasons and the time of day.

Dr. Tan's Strategy of Twelve Magical Points

The two rotating fish of the Tai Ji represent an active, global equilibrium between the yin and yang attributes. The yang emerges, increases, reaches its highest peak and recedes. Then yin emerges, increases, reaches its highest peak and recedes. Without the yin, there is no yang; without the yang, there is no yin. The two dots within the Tai Ji symbol suggest that the seed of the opposite energy is contained at the extreme point of each of the two forces. This alternating energetic rotation is a natural movement of opposite forces that can be utilized to create change in physical, mental or emotional conditions.

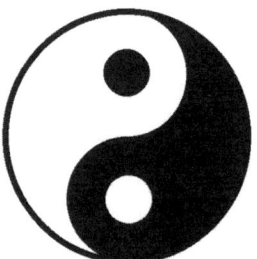

Tai Ji Symbol

To draft a treatment strategy based on the Five Systems, an alternating format of selected yin and yang meridians create the Yin/Yang Balancing Dynamic. As demonstrated below, the yin meridian on the upper right attracts the yang meridian on the upper left. This yang meridian attracts the yin on the lower left limb. Then the lower left yin attracts the lower right yang. The connection is completed with the lower right yang attracting the upper right yin.

Yin/Yang Balancing Dynamic

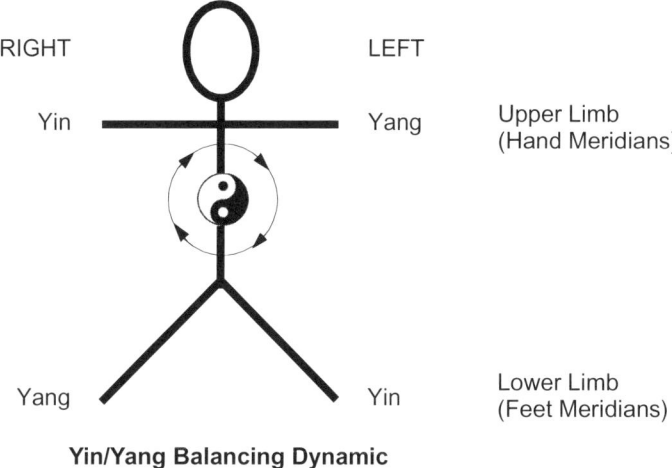

Yin/Yang Balancing Dynamic

The format can be reversed so that the yin and yang are on opposite sides of the body. If a point strategy is found to produce improvement for a condition, inverting the point format every other treatment is suggested. Reversing sides may also prove more beneficial if ashi points indicate a particular side.

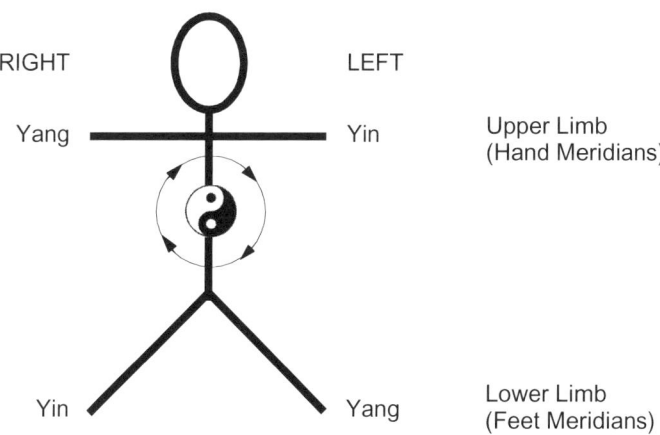

Yin/Yang Balancing Dynamic (Reversed Sides)

Dr. Tan's Strategy of Twelve Magical Points

As shown by the arrows on the figures, the mutual attraction between the yin and yang meridians generates an alternating energetic rotation analogous to the dynamic balance represented in the Tai Ji symbol. Consider how kinetic energy is generated by a bicycle rider. The continuous rotation of the wheels creates the necessary speed and momentum to keep the bicycle balanced and moving forward. The same logic of kinetic energy can be applied to the dynamic balance of the Tai Ji symbol. The force created by the attraction of polar opposites, yin and yang, shifts the body from a state of imbalance to a state of balance. Using one of the Five Systems on the Yin/Yang Balancing Format is a powerful strategy for creating equilibrium in the body.

To set up a treatment strategy, first determine the sick meridian(s). Then apply the Five Systems to select additional meridians to be needled in addition to the sick meridian. For example, a patient presents with nausea. The two primary meridians to consider as the sick meridians are Stomach and Pericardium because of their meridian relationships to the location of discomfort. System 2 (the Bie-Jing System) and System 4 (Chinese Clock Opposites) both balance the Yang Ming and Jue Yin channels. Having chosen one hand yin meridian and one foot yang meridian, we again look to the Five Systems to choose our remaining hand yang meridian and foot yin meridian to complete the dynamic balance. The Spleen and San Jiao meridians are also balanced by System 4. These choices are reinforced by System 3 (the Biao-Li or Interior/Exterior System) with San Jiao balancing Pericardium and Spleen balancing Stomach. These harmonizing components create a strongly reinforced dynamic balance.

Point location is initially determined by the primary meridian selected. In this case, the primary meridian is Stomach. The affected area is around the Stomach organ located on the trunk.

Yin/Yang Balancing Dynamic

Using the Imaging Format, the trunk can be superimposed on the leg and the umbilicus pictured at the level of the knee. The location of the nausea is about one-third of the distance between the navel and the top of the shoulders. If the image of the leg is reversed, ST36 is the appropriate point. If the same distance above the knee at ST34 is more ashi, then this reversed image is more appropriate than ST36. SP9 is a mirrored point to ST36. PC6 and SJ5 are both Luo-Connecting points and therefore produce a stronger bond between the pairs of points.

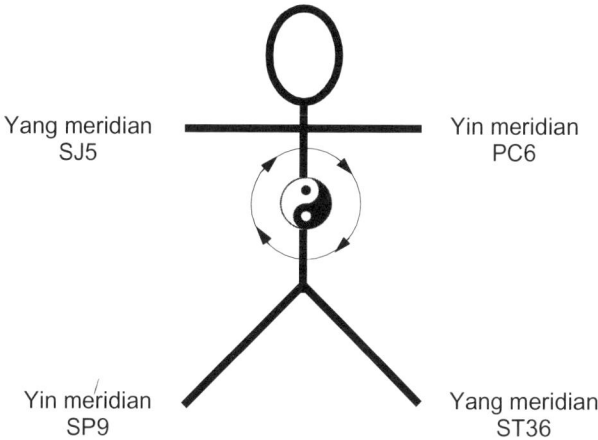

**Yin/Yang Balancing Format for
Dr. Tan's Treatment of Common Stomach Disorders**

The Yin/Yang Balancing Dynamic principle is best applied in acupuncture treatment strategy to treat conditions with no significant localized pain, or for pain all over the body in multiple meridians. For this reason, if a patient only presents with elbow pain, the best results usually occur from simply needling one limb. The Yin/Yang balancing dynamic need not be applied in these cases. Rather, diseases with symptoms affecting the whole body such as chronic fatigue, nausea, insomnia, emphysema and menopause are most efficiently treated using this format.

Dr. Tan's Strategy of Twelve Magical Points

For example, if a patient presents with only right-sided knee pain at KI10, check for ashi points on the meridians suggested by the Five Systems applying the Mirroring or Imaging Formats. All four limbs do not necessarily need to be needled. If the left side is more ashi at HT3, then a few needles around HT3 (or only HT3) are sufficient for a successful treatment.

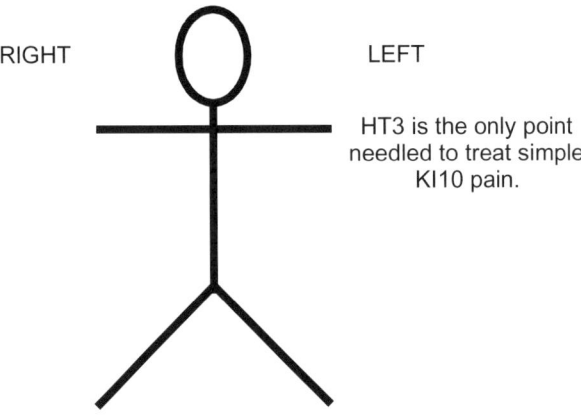

Format for One-Limb Treatment

The Yin/Yang Balancing Format is extremely effective whether an imbalance is external or internal, cold or hot, excess or deficient, pain related or non-pain related. The patient often easily relaxes and falls asleep while the body actively shifts into the state of balance. Depending on the condition, initial treatments may need to be repeated two to three times per week until the symptoms do not return until the day of the next treatment.

BALANCE METHOD TREATMENT GUIDELINES

The previous chapters include all of the necessary ingredients to organize a Balance Method treatment. The Guidelines listed below are a step-by-step procedure to assist in the process of creating a treatment strategy. Questions about treatments may be addressed to Dr. Tan at *drtan@earthlink.net*, or the online Forum at *www.drtanshow.com*.

1. Ask questions, listen, observe and palpate.
2. Determine the sick meridian at the site of the complaint.
3. Palpate areas that mirror or image the complaint site.
4. Choose the needled meridian(s) to balance the sick meridian(s) based on the Five Systems, the Twelve Points Strategy or another Advanced System.
5. Select points using the Mirroring Format, Imaging Format, Four-Segment Timing or an Advanced System.
6. Arrange points on the Yin/Yang Balancing Dynamic if applicable.
7. Get "Da" chi with each needle.
8. Retain needles 45-90 minutes.
9. Stimulate the needles at least once during the treatment.
10. Arrange initial treatment plan with treatments two to three times per week. Reduce treatment frequency as the patient improves.

Dr. Tan's Strategy of Twelve Magical Points

PART TWO:
The Strategy of Twelve Magical Points

The Concept	45
The Mechanics	47
The Patterns	57
Case Studies	71

THE CONCEPT

The Five Systems of the Balance Method are used most effectively when the sick meridian is identifiable. However, idiopathic disorders such as fibromyalgia, chronic fatigue syndrome and irritable bowel syndrome are increasingly common in modern practice. Many of these pathologies do not present with pain or numbness in a particular region, or the pain may extend over a broad area. For example, fibromyalgia pain may move to different areas or spread over the entire body; consequently, it is difficult to determine specific sick meridians since many or all of the meridians are involved.

In addition, more and more patients are complaining of headaches, insomnia, allergies, anxiety and depression. Often, complicated cases simultaneously involve numerous conditions such as: migraines with insomnia and depression, chronic fatigue syndrome with allergies and anxiety, or repetitive motion injury with irritable bowel syndrome. These conditions involving multiple and/or ambiguous meridians prove most challenging for an acupuncturist who relies on meridian theory for diagnosis and treatment strategy. The Strategy of Twelve Magical Points was designed to treat complicated pathological conditions with exceptional clinical efficacy.

> *This revolutionary technique combines the*
> *Five Transporting Points, the 12 main meridians,*
> *the Imaging Format, Four-Segment Timing and*
> *the Yin/Yang Balancing Dynamic.*

Dr. Tan's Strategy of Twelve Magical Points

THE MECHANICS

Overview

All twelve meridians are used in the *Strategy of Twelve Magical Points* because the affected area may involve several channels or may not be identifiable. A group of three points are used on each limb, for a total of 12 points. Each group contains three individual meridians with the same yin/yang attribute. The groups are each composed of three Shu-Transporting points which cover a particular anatomical region on each limb. By using these points, the whole body is treated under the Imaging Format. The groups are chosen based on their relationship to Four-Segment Timing, and therefore a cyclical rhythm is created which brings the body into balance. The points are then arranged on the Yin/Yang Balancing Dynamic in a Tai Ji pattern. This further sets the treatment into motion and shifts the body from a state of imbalance to balance. The following six sections will breakdown all the necessary ingredients for constructing a treatment using the *Strategy of Twelve Magical Points*. Then all of the ingredients will be put together in a step-by-step format, and each of the 16 possible patterns will be clearly illustrated. Finally, case studies will assist readers in the practical application of the strategy.

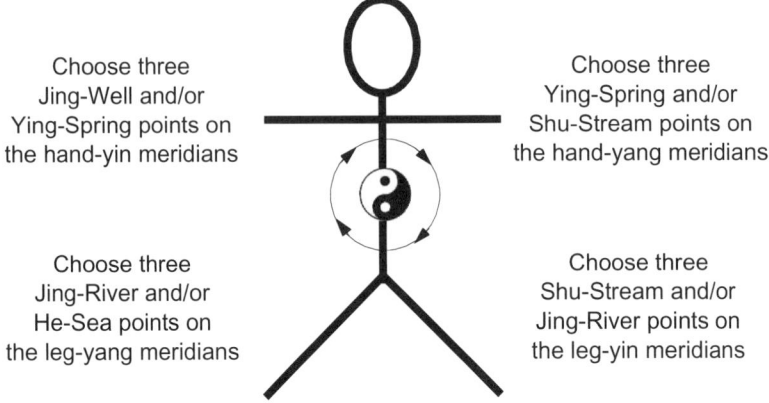

Example of Twelve Points Strategy Layout

1. The Five Shu-Transporting Points

The ancient classics of Chinese Medicine contain various theories concerning the significance of the Five Shu-Transporting Points. The *Classic of Difficulties* explains the association of the Transporting Points with the Five Elements: wood, fire, earth, metal and water. The *Nan Jing* discusses the energetic dynamic and function of each Transporting Point: well, gushing, transporting, traversing and uniting.

Among other clinical applications, the *Spiritual Axis* defines the tonifying and draining functions of each Shu point based on mother-son relationships. All of these philosophies can be used alone to produce impressive treatment strategies. However, faster and more effective results can be achieved by combining these existing theories with the *Strategy of Twelve Magical Points*. A review of these points is found in the following chart.

The Mechanics

	Jing Well	Ying Spring	Shu Stream	Jing River	He Sea
UPPER LIMB					
Yin					
Lung	LU11	LU10	LU9	LU8	LU5
Pericardium	PC9	PC8	PC7	PC5	PC3
Heart	HT9	HT8	HT7	HT4	HT3
Yang					
Large Intestine	LI1	LI2	LI3	LI5	LI11
San Jiao	SJ1	SJ2	SJ3	SJ6	SJ10
Small Intestine	SI1	SI2	SI3	SI5	SI8
LOWER LIMB					
Yin					
Spleen	SP1	SP2	SP3	SP5	SP9
Liver	LV1	LV2	LV3	LV4	LV8
Kidney	KI1	KI2	KI3	KI7	KI10
Yang					
Stomach	ST45	ST44	ST43	ST41	ST36
Gall Bladder	GB44	GB43	GB41	GB38	GB34
Urinary Bladder	UB67	UB66	UB65	UB60	UB40

Anatomical Distribution of Five Shu Points

Dr. Tan's Strategy of Twelve Magical Points

2. Meridian Selection

All 12 meridians are always used in the strategy. One upper-limb set covers the three hand-yin meridians, while the other upper-limb set covers the three hand-yang meridians. Likewise, one lower-limb set covers the three leg-yin meridians, while the other lower-limb set covers the three leg-yang meridians.

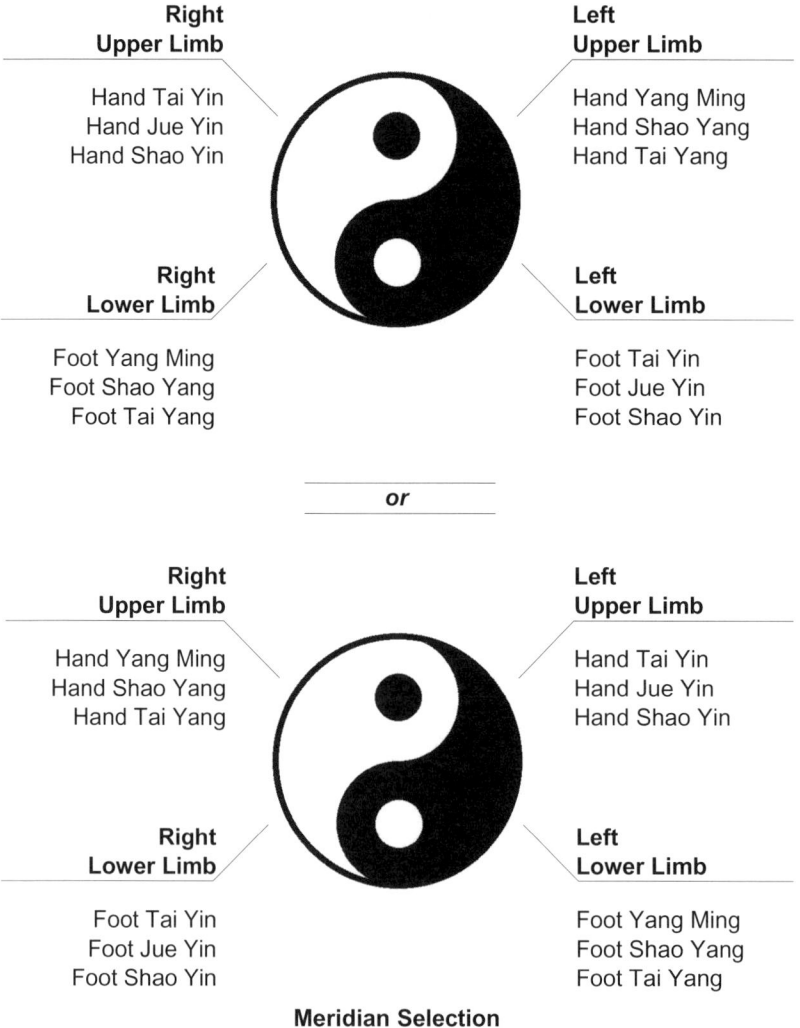

Meridian Selection

The Mechanics

3. Imaging Format

The next level of balance is accomplished by applying the Imaging Format to the anatomical regions covered by the Five Shu Points. Each region reflects a different area of the body beginning with the Jing-Well points at the tips of the fingers and toes, and concluding with the He-Sea points at the knees and elbows. In essence, the whole body is treated when you utilize the Five Shu Points.

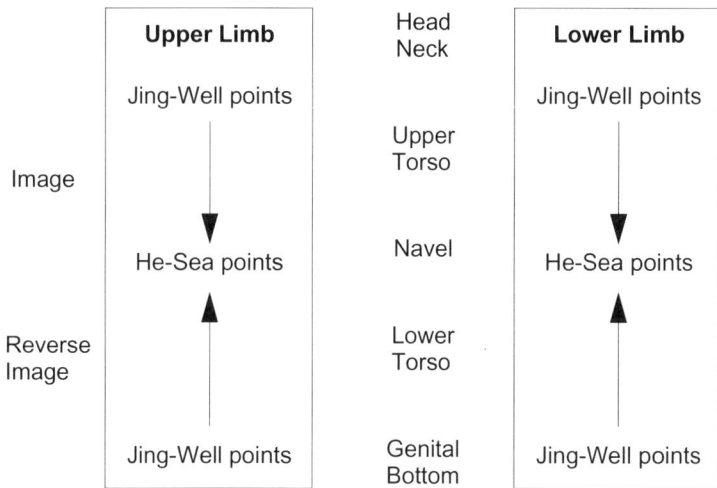

Application of Five Shu Points to Imaging Format

Dr. Tan's Strategy of Twelve Magical Points

4. Four-Segment Timing

The Five Shu Points are arranged into categories: Jing-Well, Ying-Spring, Shu-Stream, Jing-River and He-Sea. As discussed earlier, these five categories share segments from the Four-Segment Timing. Each limb represents one of the 4 segments, and therefore each limb may contain Shu points from 2 categories.

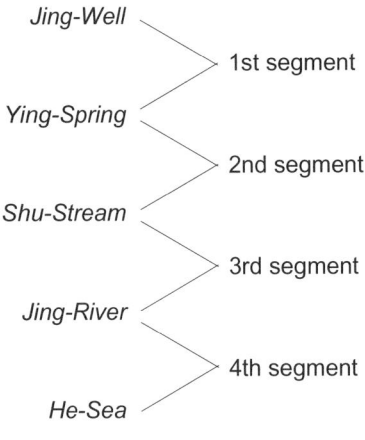

Four-Segment Timing

The Mechanics

5. Yin/Yang Balancing Dynamic

The basic Yin/Yang Balancing Dynamic serves as a model to format the points.

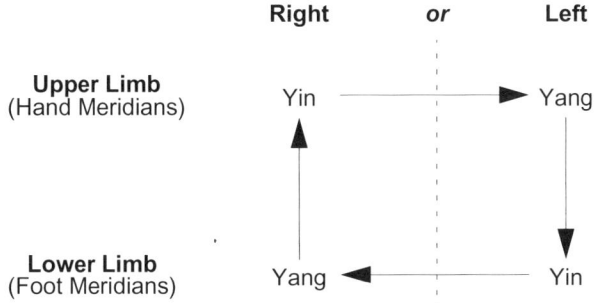

Basic Yin/Yang Dynamic Balancing Format

The four groups of points alternate in a yin-yang-yin-yang format.

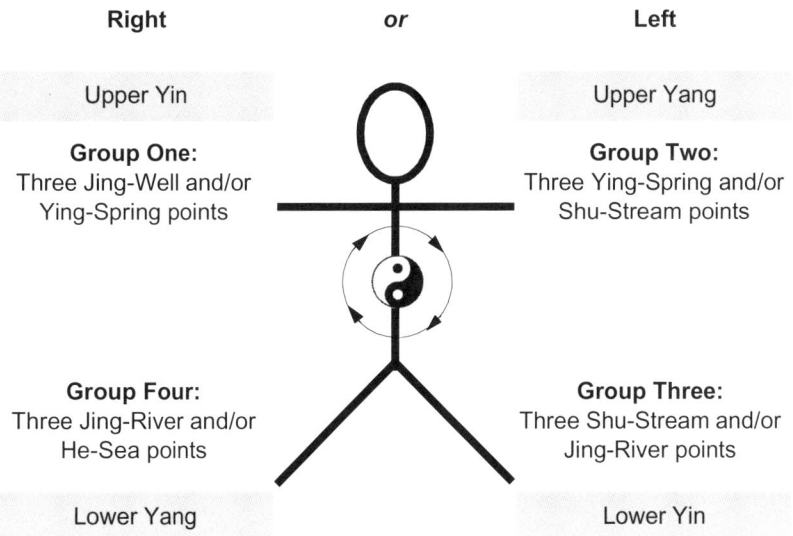

Yin/Yang Dynamic Balancing Format With Group Arrangement

6. Mirroring Format

Points can be selected and arranged to reflect anatomical regions of the body by application of the Mirroring Format. For example, if a patient's chief complaint is peripheral neuropathy in the Jing-Well/Ying-Spring area on the left foot, Patterns 1 and 2 are considered due to the Mirroring Format. Both of these patterns begin with yin Jing-Well/Ying-Spring points (Segment 1) on the upper right arm which addresses the left foot. In this case, look for other symptoms to refine your pattern selection. If the patient also suffers right knee pain on the yang channels, then Pattern 2 clearly is the best choice because of the upper left yang He-Sea points.

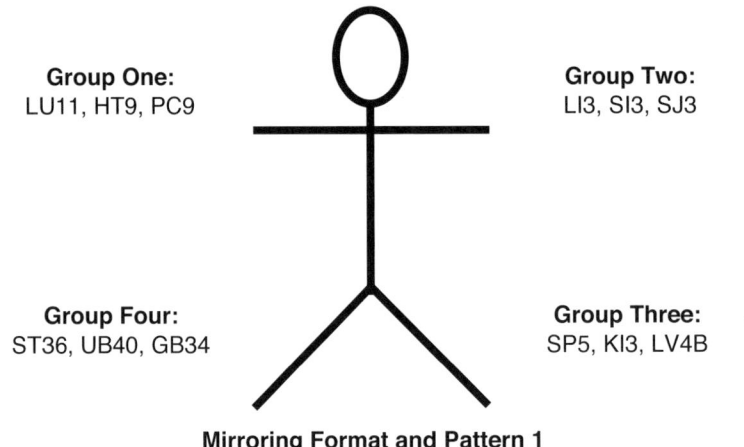

Group One:
LU11, HT9, PC9

Group Two:
LI3, SI3, SJ3

Group Four:
ST36, UB40, GB34

Group Three:
SP5, KI3, LV4B

Mirroring Format and Pattern 1

The Mechanics
Step-by-Step Guidelines to Constructing a Treatment

1. Three individual meridians with the same yin/yang attribute are chosen for each limb. These four sets utilize all 12 meridians. The sets are formatted in an alternating Yin/Yang Balancing Dynamic.

   Example:
   Right arm: LU, HT, PC
   Left arm: LI, SI, SJ
   Left leg: SP, KD, LV
   Right leg: ST, UB, GB

2. Each set of 3 meridians represents one segment from the Four-Segment Timing chart. You may begin Segment 1 on any of the four limbs.

   Example:
   Right arm: LU, HT, PC (Segment 1)
   Left arm: LI, SI, SJ (Segment 2)
   Left leg: SP, KD, LV (Segment 3)
   Right leg: ST, UB, GB (Segment 4)

3. Choose Shu-Transporting points for each set which correspond with the associated segment. You may choose to use only one group of Shu points for a particular set, or a combination of the two groups. For example, segment one is composed of Jing-Well and Ying-Spring points. You may choose to use 3 Jing-Well points or 3 Ying-Spring points, or a combination of both Jing-Well and Ying-Spring points.

   Example:
   Right arm: LU 11, HT 9, PC 9 (all Jing-Well points) *or*
   　　　　　　LU 10, HT 8, PC 8 (all Ying-Spring points) *or*
   　　　　　　LU 10, HT 9, PC 8 (any combo of Jing-Well and Ying-Spring points)

Dr. Tan's Strategy of Twelve Magical Points

4. The segments follow the sequential ascent of the 5 Shu Points, starting with the Jing-Well points and ending with the He-Sea points. This creates a dynamic balance where the qi moves from limb to limb in the same manner as it would ascend from the Jing-Well to the He-Sea. This continuous movement represents the body in motion when applied to the Imaging Format.

   Example:
   Right arm: LU 11, HT8, PC 9 (Segment 1)
   Left arm: LI3, SI3, SJ3 (Segment 2)
   Left leg: SP5, KD3, LV4 (Segment 3)
   Right leg: ST36, UB 40, GB40 (Segment 4)

5. A variety of combinations are possible depending on which limb you choose for the start of your treatment, the clockwise or counterclockwise direction of your treatment, and the particular combination of Shu points that are chosen for each limb. The next section will outline each of the 16 possible patterns that are used as the framework for your treatment. You may choose a pattern which allows you to focus on specific imbalances in your individual patient. The Imaging and Mirroring Formats will help in your selection on a case-by-case basis.

   Example: Fibromyalgia pain with left-sided Yang Ming elbow pain.

   In this case, you could combine the *Strategy of Twelve Magical Points* (for overall fibromyalgia pain) with System 1 of the Balance Method (for elbow pain). Therefore, you already know that you want to end your treatment with needles around ST 36 on the right leg. For this reason, you may choose Pattern 1 which begins with yin Jing-Well points on the right arm and ends with yang He-Sea points on the right leg.

THE PATTERNS

The Eight Patterns

The Eight Patterns of the Twelve Points Strategy follow three basic rules:

1. The sequential direction of a pattern always begins with Groups of Shu-Transportings points from Segment 1, moves to Segment 2, then Segment 3 and finally ends with Segment 4. Therefore, you always begin with Jing-Well points and end with He-Sea points.

2. You may choose to begin on any limb, and you may move in a clockwise or a counterclockwise direction.

3. You may start with a group of yin meridians, or you may start with a group of yang meridians.

For example, Pattern 1 begins with yin Jing-Well and/or Ying-Spring points on the upper right, and moves to yang Ying-Spring and/or Shu-Stream on the upper left (clockwise direction). The sequence of Pattern 2 also begins with yin Jing-Well and/or Ying-Spring points on the upper right, but then

Dr. Tan's Strategy of Twelve Magical Points

moves to yang Ying-Spring and/or Shu-Stream on the lower right (counterclockwise direction). In Pattern 3, the sequence begins with yang Jing-Well points on the upper right and moves to yin Shu-Stream points on the upper left (clockwise direction).

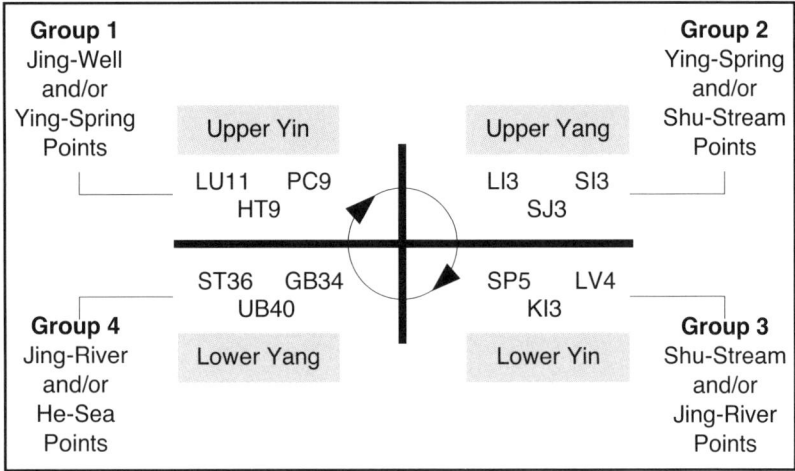

Format for Pattern 1

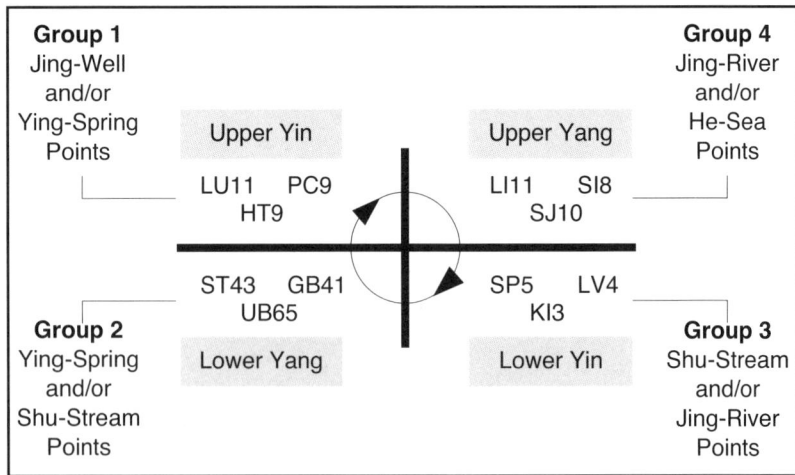

Format for Pattern 2

The Patterns

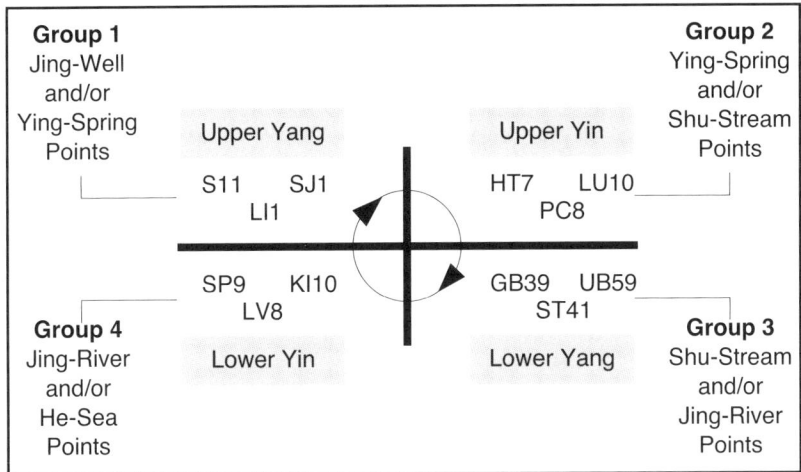

Format for Pattern 3

Flipping the Point Sequence to the Opposite Side of the Body

Each of the Eight Patterns may be flipped to the opposite side of the body which creates a total of sixteen possible patterns. Points on the right side of the body move directly to the left side of the body and vice versa. These flipped patterns are referred to as "f" patterns in the illustrations. The "f" patterns always move in the opposite direction of the original pattern in order to maintain sequential order.

For example, Pattern 1 begins with yin Jing-Well and/or Ying-Spring points on the upper right, and moves to yang Ying-Spring and/or Shu-Stream on the upper left. It moves from segment to segment in a clockwise direction. Pattern 1f is composed of the same points as the original pattern. However, it begins with yin Jing-Well and/or Ying-Spring points on the upper left, and moves to yang Ying-Spring and/or Shu-Stream on the upper right. It moves from segment to segment in a counterclockwise direction.

Dr. Tan's Strategy of Twelve Magical Points

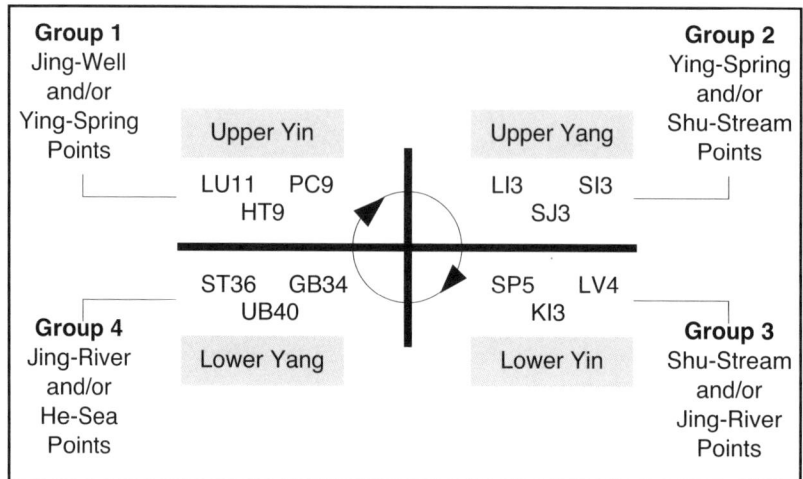

Pattern 1

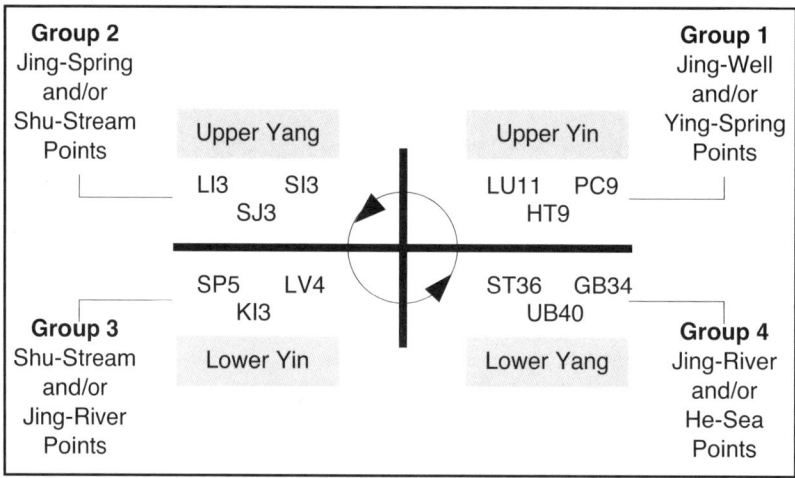

Pattern 1f—Flipping the Pattern

The eight "flipped" patterns provide additional treatment choices which may allow the practitioner to tailor a treatment for specific complaints. For example, consider a patient presenting with peripheral neuropathy of the right large toe and right-sided elbow pain at SJ10. Pattern 1f specifically would fit

The Patterns

this case because the upper Jing-Well points and lower He-Sea points are both on the left side. This combines the Twelve Points Strategy, System 1 and the Mirroring Format.

Dr. Tan's Strategy of Twelve Magical Points

Pattern 1

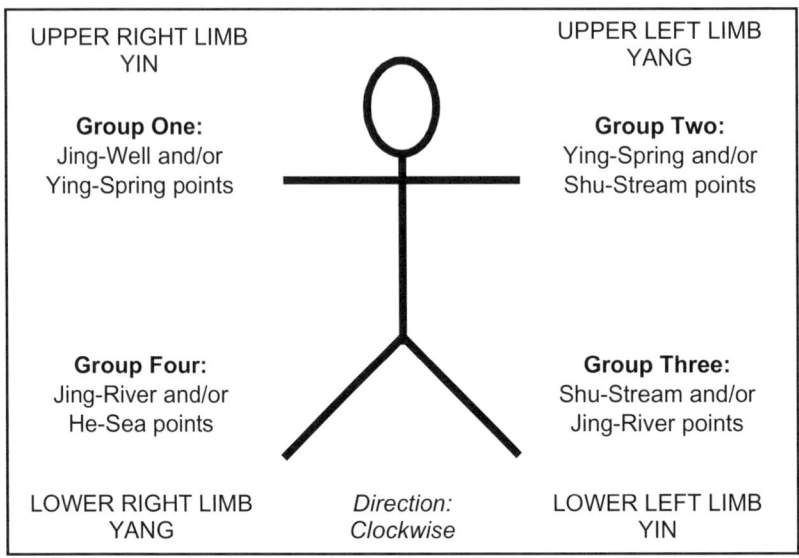

Pattern 1

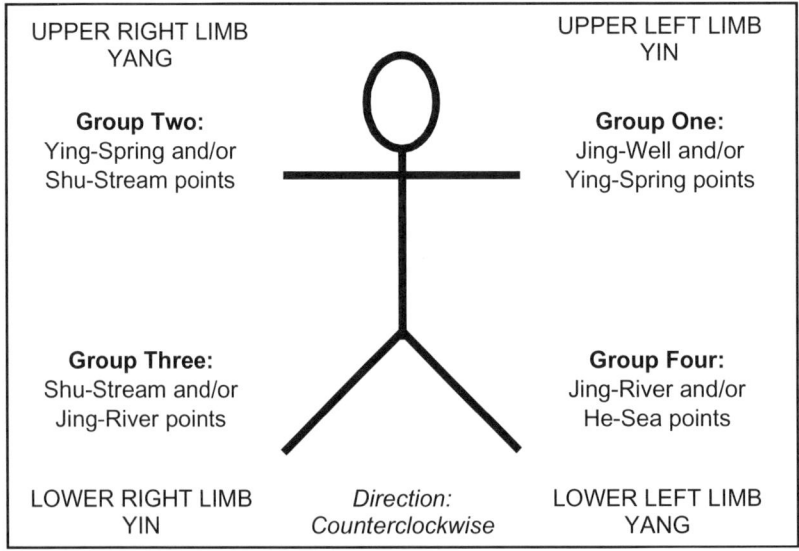

Pattern 1f

The Patterns

Pattern 2

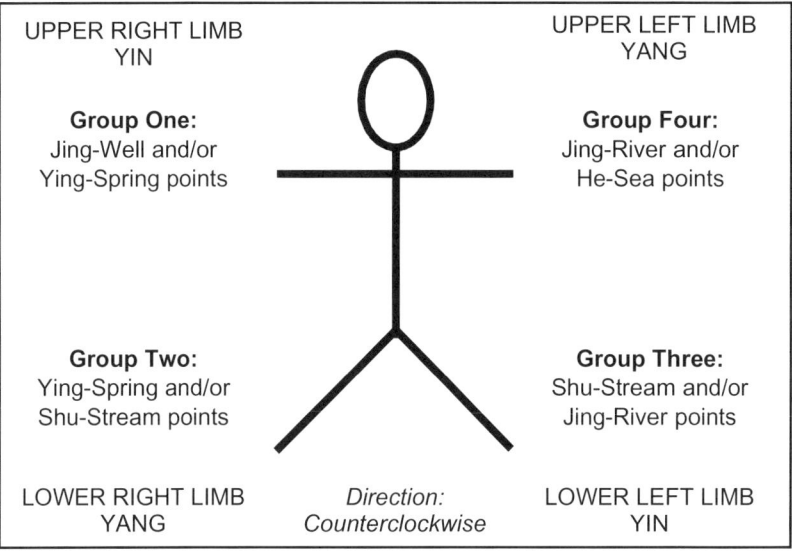

Pattern 2

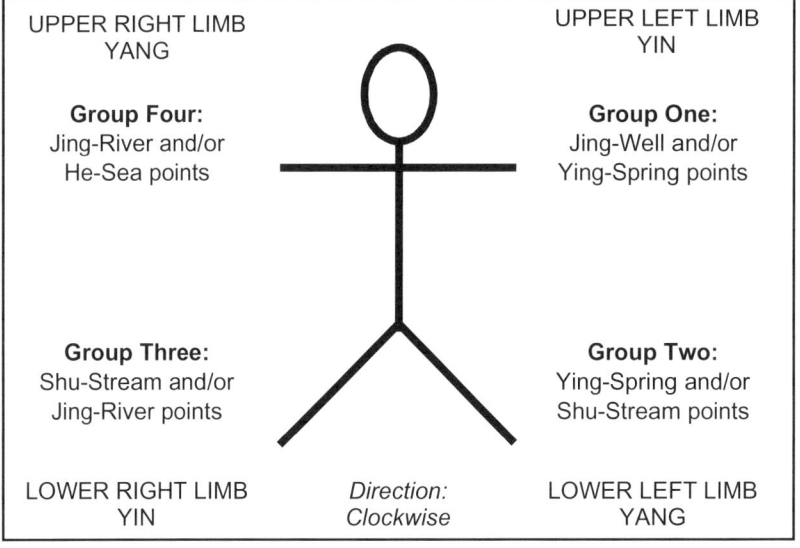

Pattern 2f

Dr. Tan's Strategy of Twelve Magical Points

Pattern 3

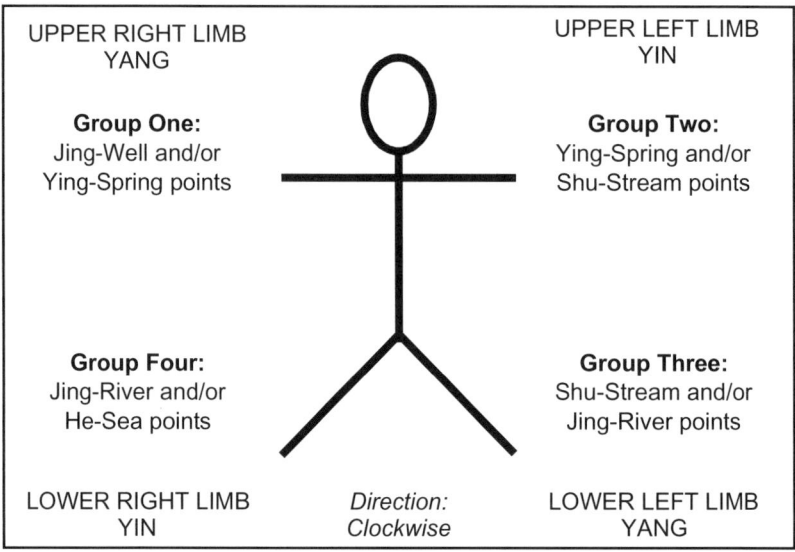

Pattern 3

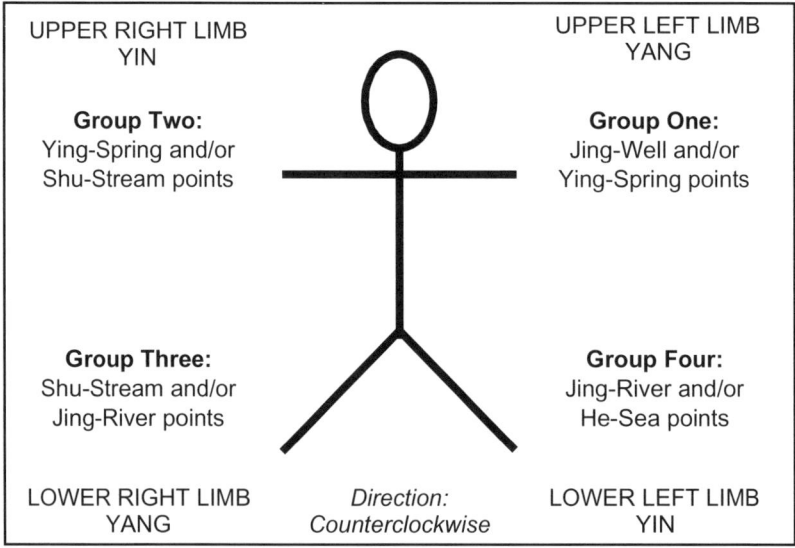

Pattern 3f

The Patterns

Pattern 4

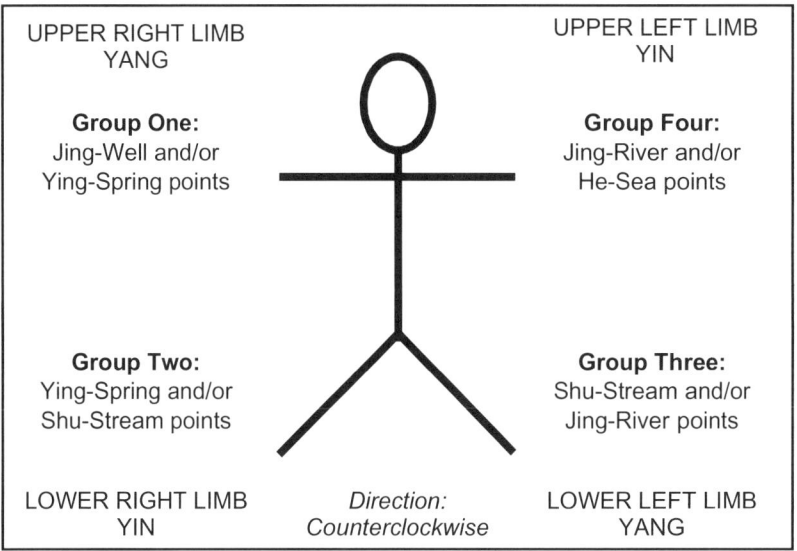

Pattern 4

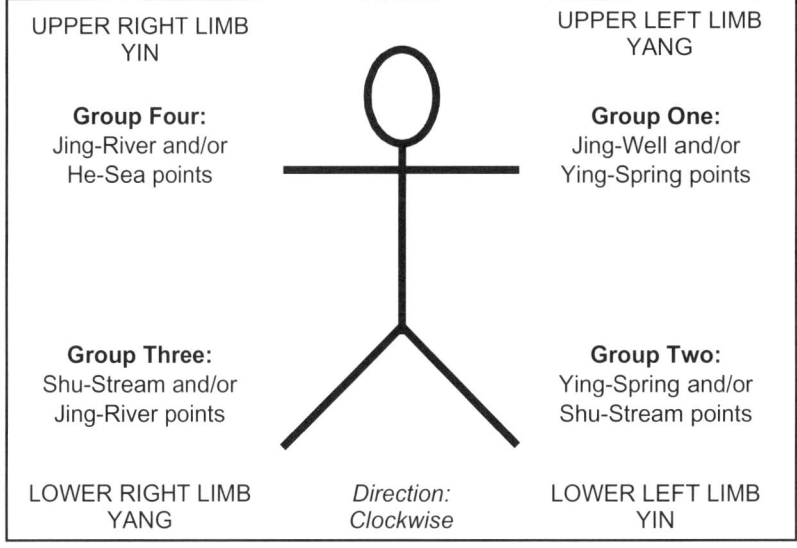

Pattern 4f

Pattern 5

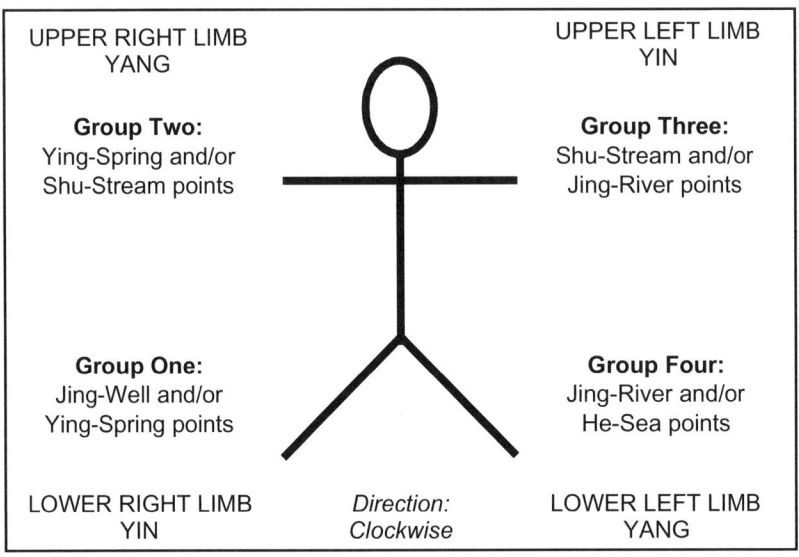

Pattern 5

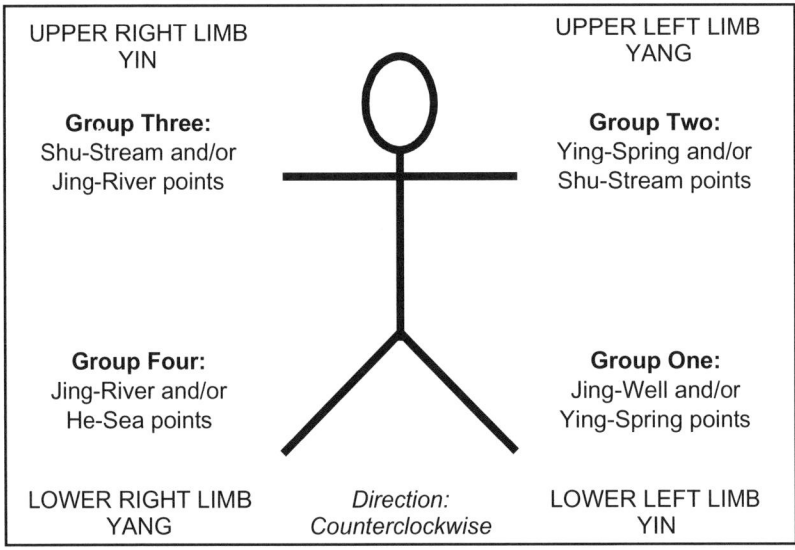

Pattern 5f

The Patterns

Pattern 6

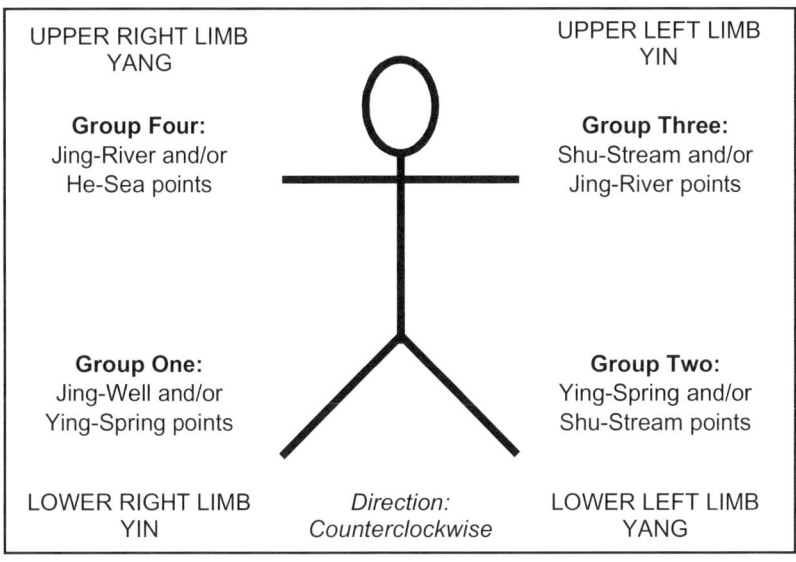

Pattern 6

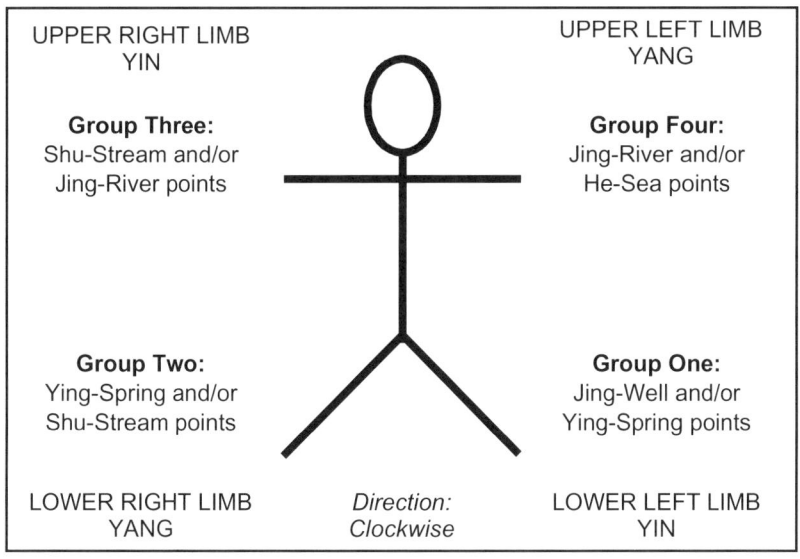

Pattern 6f

Pattern 7

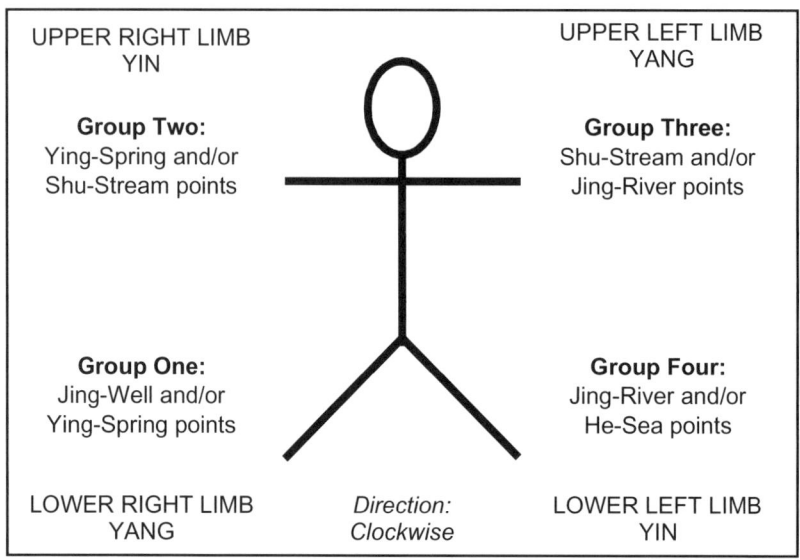

Pattern 7

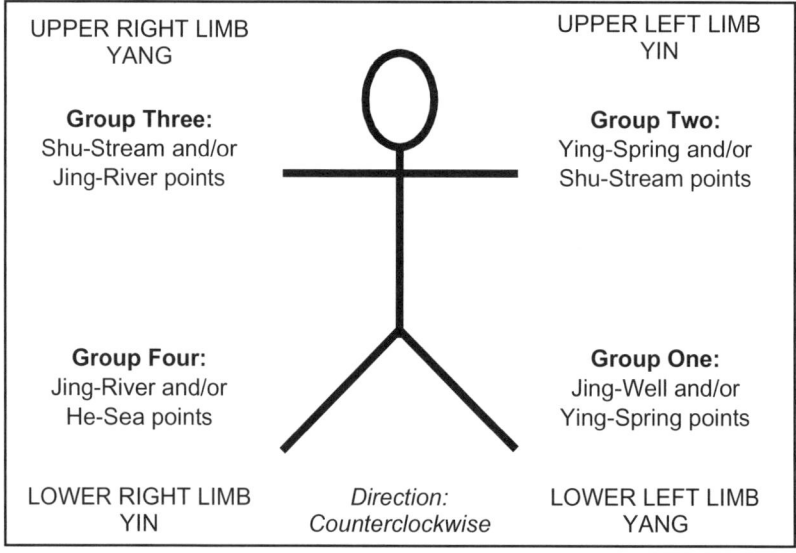

Pattern 7f

The Patterns

Pattern 8

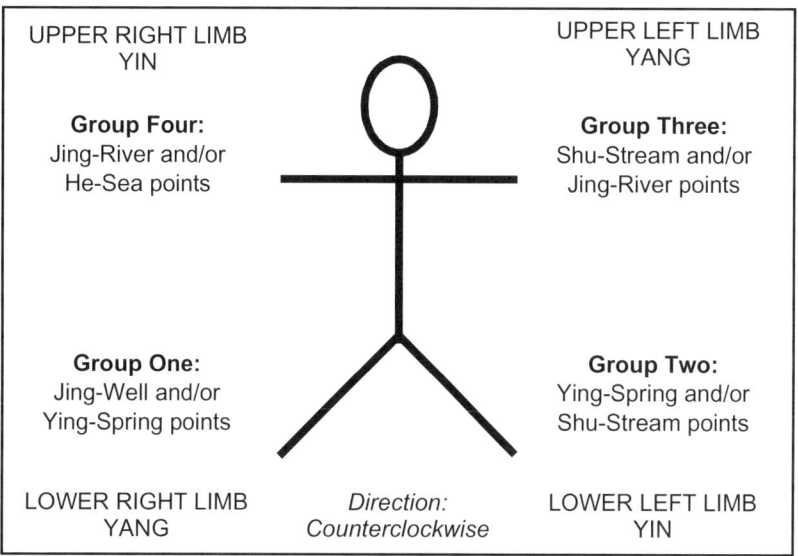

Pattern 8

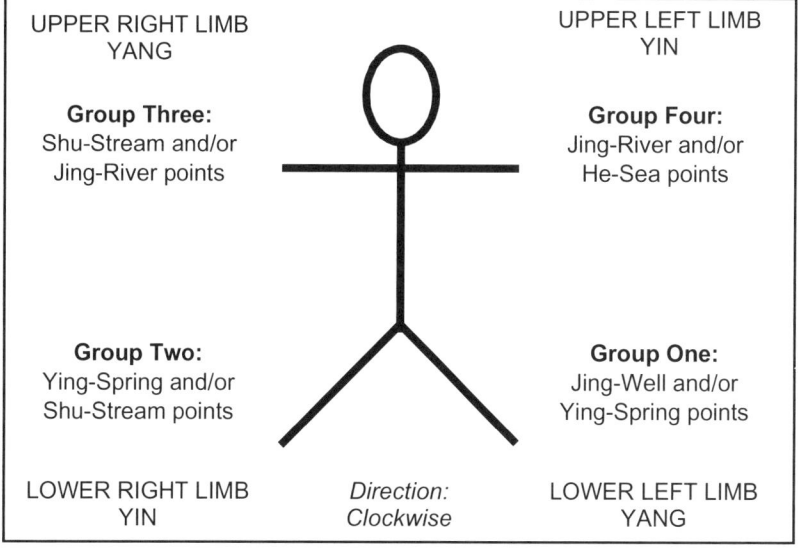

Pattern 8f

Dr. Tan's Strategy of Twelve Magical Points

CASE STUDIES

———•———

The following case studies were chosen from the countless patients who have been treated successfully with the Strategy of Twelve Magical Points. The cases serve to assist the reader in understanding the logic behind pattern selection. While the preceding sections have focused on the mechanics of the strategy, the following examples will demonstrate the practical application. The method is called a "strategy" because it is reveals an innovative approach to applying classical acupuncture theory. This book should not serve as a technical manual in which the practitioner follows specific points based on empirical data. Rather, it provides the necessary concepts for designing personalized treatment prescriptions. Therefore, the case studies will reveal that there are no exact "rules" to the strategy. The idea behind this method is to utilize successive segments on distal portions of the limbs. These segments cover all the anatomical regions necessary to create an image of the body from head to foot. For this reason, Yuan-Source, Luo-Connecting and Xi-Cleft points may be used in your treatments because they are located among the anatomical regions covered by the Shu-Transporting points. As an example, LI4 (Yuan-Source point) may be substituted for LI3 (Shu-Stream point) because it still serves to image the anatomical region covered by Segment 2. In addition, the cases will also demonstrate the importance of adjusting treatments based on patient feedback. Often, the original pattern and the "flipped" pattern may need to be alternated to achieve the best results. Overall, the most effective treatments will arise out of the practitioner's own creativity and flexibility when applying the ideas behind this strategy.

PATTERN 1

SLEEPLESS AND STRESSED IN SAN DIEGO

Morey, 56, was slightly overweight and had suffered with severe migraines for two years. His headaches began after his company down-sized and became part of a larger corporation. He lay awake every night and worried about his family's future. When his headaches first began, Morey went to a medical doctor and got strong medication. The pills did not help, and the pain was so bad that he could not sleep. The most intense headaches could continue for up to three days, and finally Morey decided to try acupuncture as a last resort.

Morey's pain was located at the occipital, frontal and temporal areas of his head. Often, the pain would move around or cover his entire head. On his first visit, he complained of a left-sided headache behind his eyeball, covering the Gall Bladder and San Jiao meridians. Therefore, the Shao Yang meridians were treated using the Balance Method. However, the headache moved to the top of his head during the treatment, rendering the Shao Yang treatment no longer applicable. The Strategy of Twelve Magical Points was then chosen to cover numerous channels. Within seconds of needle insertion, the headache pain changed quality to a wavelike pattern. The intensity of the pain

Case Studies

fluctuated and then slowly decreased. Bilateral Ear Shen Men was added to calm him down and help his insomnia. He was encouraged to relax and sleep if possible.

Thirty minutes later, the intensity of the pain lessened by 80%. The needles were stimulated again. Forty-five minutes later, Morey was released with no headache. The initial treatment plan was three times per week. During the first week, he experienced some reoccurrence, but the intensity of pain was greatly reduced. After three more treatments, Morey had experienced only one headache lasting two hours, and the pain was 75% less than the previous migraines.

By the third week, treatments were reduced to two times per week. During this week, he experienced only one headache that lasted an hour and disappeared after a nap. He was no longer taking pain medication and was sleeping soundly through most nights. To stabilize the result, two treatments per week for two weeks were recommended. Morey was released in less than two months. His two-year problem was completely resolved by Pattern 1.

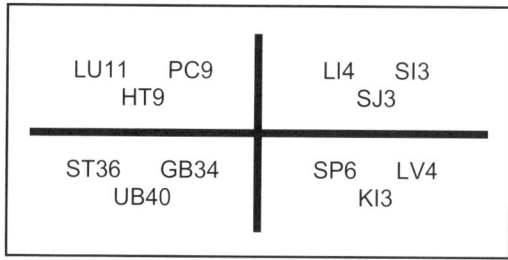

Pattern 1

PATTERNS 1 AND 1F
TRAVELS WITH RUTHEY

Ruthey, 48, complained of insomnia and generalized muscle pain. She had been diagnosed with chronic fatigue syndrome and fibromyalgia. Frequent business trips took her away from home each week. The years of travel depleted her energy and aggravated the pain. Yet, Ruthey was determined to provide for her children's college education, and she wanted to work hard so that she could retire early.

Often the pain started with a headache and then moved to the rest of her body. She could not pinpoint exactly where the pain was located, and all 12 meridians seemed to be involved. Pattern 1 was selected because yin Jing-Well points on the hands are very effective for headaches, while LV4 and SI3 treat scapula and neck pain. The initial treatment plan was three times per week for six weeks.

Ruthey noticed significant improvement during the first week. On a pain scale from 1-10, her body pain was reduced from a level 10 to a level 3-4. Her headaches disappeared, her insomnia decreased and she had more energy. However, her improvement was at a standstill by the fourth treatment. At this point, Pattern 1f was chosen. Ruthey continued to improve and her pain disappeared over the treatment period.

During the sixth week, she traveled to Europe for one week. The interruption in treatment was a good test to see how well she would maintain her improvement without acupuncture. Although her travel schedule was heavy, she remained pain free. To stabilize the results, Ruthey came for treatment one to two times per week for four more weeks and was released with no pain.

Case Studies

LU11 PC9 HT9	LI4 SI3 SJ3
ST36 GB34 UB40	SP6 LV4 KI3

LI4 SI3 SJ3	LU11 PC9 HT9
SP6 LV4 KI3	ST36 GB34 UB40

Patterns 1 and 1f

PATTERN 1

HAROLD'S ALTERNATING OBSTRUCTION

Harold was a heavyset man in his late thirties. He had a genuine interest in alternative medicine and took yoga classes several times a month.

He complained that the left side of his trunk and left knee felt "blocked" for two months with no apparent reason. He reported a feeling of stagnation that was not relieved by yoga or other energetic exercises. Harold decided to seek treatment when the sensation of obstruction began to alternate between the right and left sides of his body.

He also complained of fullness in the middle burner with bloating and some food retention. His blood pressure was within normal range and his pulse showed no irregular beats. There was no redness or swelling in the affected areas.

The Strategy of Twelve Magical Points was chosen because no particular meridians were affected in this case. The He-Sea points in Pattern 1 can image the middle jiao and also treat left-sided knee pain. The first two acupuncture treatments were given on consecutive days because Harold lived 100 miles from the clinic. A friend allowed him to spend the night in order to get two acupuncture treatments. After the first treatment, he felt 80% better. The second treatment cleared up the residual discomfort. Two weeks later, Harold sent a letter of appreciation stating that he felt great and had no more discomfort.

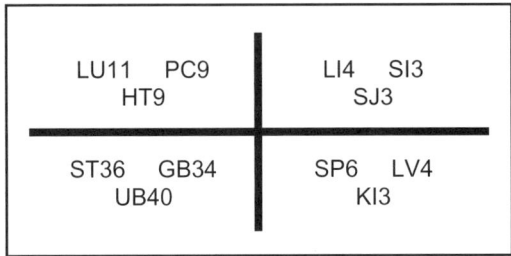

Pattern 1

PATTERN 2

TOP O' THE MORNIN'

George, 65, was a European gentleman with a grandfatherly kindness. He always had a good sense of humor despite physical discomfort. He suffered from occasional headaches, abdominal pain, alternating loose stools and constipation, gas and right-sided knee pain. The knee pain covered the entire knee and therefore a specific meridian could not be identified. The lower abdominal pain wrapped around his torso and indicated involvement of the Dai Mai channel (Eight Extra Meridian). The pulse was wiry, and the left guan and cun positions felt weak.

Pattern 2 was selected because the He-Sea points on the left elbow could treat his right-sided knee pain, digestive disorders and headaches. In addition, GB41 (master point of the Dai Channel) addressed his abdominal pain. The initial treatment

Case Studies

plan was twice per week for four weeks. After the first treatment, the abdominal pain and headaches were 70% better and his knee pain improved by 50%.

Over the treatment period, all of George's symptoms stabilized. The knee pain was 95% gone and the headaches disappeared. George was sleeping well and his energy increased. The discomfort in the Dai channel was gone and his stools normalized, yet he continued to have flatulence. At this time, the pulse felt weak in both guan positions.

```
        LU11  PC9    |  LI11  SJ10
           HT9       |     SI8
   ------------------+------------------
        ST43  GB41   |  SP6  KI7
           UB65      |     LV5
```

Pattern 2

The treatment strategy was changed to the Yang Ming/Tai Yin treatment to balance digestion. This is an advanced system of the balance method that addresses internal disorders. After two weeks, his digestion greatly improved. George chose to continue treatment two times per month for energy enhancement and health maintenance.

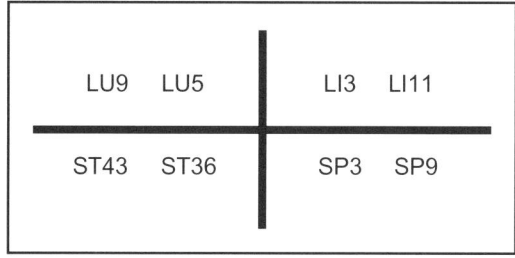

Yang Ming/Tai Yin Treatment

Dr. Tan's Strategy of Twelve Magical Points

PATTERN 2

CUTTER'S ANXIETY

Mack was a 45-year-old hairstylist with a history of Hepatitis C. He was a workaholic who had recently been under a great deal of emotional stress. Mack suffered from insomnia, headaches and pain in his right knee, left scapula and left shoulder.

Pattern 2 was chosen, along with bilateral Ear Shen Men to relieve his insomnia. Several ashi points were treated on his left leg around LV5 to treat the scapular pain. Three ashi points were needled around LI11 on the left side for the right-sided knee pain.

Seven treatments were completed within three weeks and Mack felt much better. His headaches and knee pain were gone. He still had slight shoulder pain due to repetitive use while cutting hair. During the course of the treatment, Mack also became calmer and more relaxed. Herbal medicine was dispensed to treat the fatigue associated with Hepatitis C.

LU11 PC9 HT9	LI11 SJ10 SI8
ST43 GB41 UB65	SP6 KI7 LV5

Pattern 2

PATTERN 2F

SHOPPING WITH GRANDMA

Betty was an insulin-dependent diabetic in her mid 60s. She loved to go for morning walks and excursions with her grandchildren. However, foot discomfort limited her activities and continued to worsen over time. She had burning pain in the ball of her right foot, with numbness and tingling in her toes. The pain was worst in the area of LV1 and SP1 on her right toe.

Her pulse was deep and deficient, and her tongue was red and slightly wrinkled with a scant coat. Pattern 2f was chosen because the left-sided Jing-Well points treat the right-sided toes when applying the Imaging Format. After the first treatment, the tingling and pain was greatly reduced from a level 10 to a level 4. She was very happy because she suffered with the burning pain for more than five years.

Much to her delight, she was able to go shopping with her grandchildren. The extra walking aggravated her symptoms, but the pain was not as severe as before the acupuncture treatments. Betty thought her energy improved, but she was unsure if it was due to the treatment.

After six weeks of treatments two times per week, Betty reported a 90% improvement in her symptoms and her blood sugar stabilized. She was now certain that her energy improved because she had the stamina to clean her house all day long.

Dr. Tan's Strategy of Twelve Magical Points

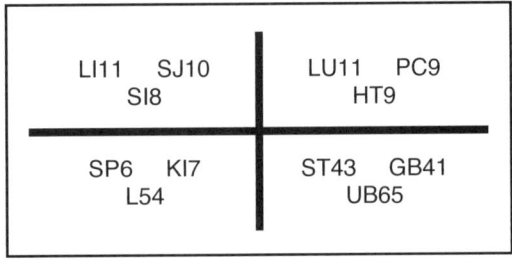

Pattern 2f

PATTERN 3F

JOEY'S VOLLEY

Joey, 39, avidly played volleyball, golf and tennis every week. At his last tournament, he landed the winning point for his volleyball team. Unfortunately, he also injured his left hand and wrist. The pain was located around SJ4 and LI5, radiating down the LI channel into LI4. Joey continued to play sports despite a western diagnosis of tendonitis.

The first phase of Joey's treatments utilized System 1 of the Balance Method. In eight treatments, the pain was stabilized using ST41, ST42, ST43 and GB40 on his right leg. He had no more pain unless he performed strenuous lifting, and therefore his treatments were reduced to once per week.

Joey then disclosed that he suffered sleeping difficulties for one year since his romantic relationship ended. He would awake at the slightest noise. In the past, Joey previously found relief from his sleeping problems by maintaining a high level of physical activity, but this was no longer the case. He also suffered from a dry mouth and bloating within an hour of eating any type of food.

Case Studies

The second treatment series combined Pattern 3f with System 1 of the Balance Method.

HT7 LU10 PC8	SI1 SJ1 LI1
GB39 UB59 UB62A ST41, 42, 43	SP9 KI10 Tan's liver point*

* Located on the medial anterior side of the condyle of the tibia bone. Look for ashi points and use oblique insertion on the bone.

Pattern 3f

Joey had three nights of uninterrupted sleep after one treatment with Pattern 3f. His stomach bloating was decreased, but his mouth was still dry. Ten treatments later, he was released symptom free. Joey receives maintenance treatments when he feels stressed.

PATTERNS 3 AND 3F

THE YOUNG CHEMIST'S FATIGUE

Fatima, 26, worked as a full-time lab assistant while attending graduate school. She had a history of Lyme disease, and now suffered with lingering fatigue and an idiopathic sore throat each morning. She also complained of depression, itchy eyes, back pain and occipital neck pain.

The chosen strategy was Pattern 3, alternating with 3f, because most of her symptoms were bilateral. This pattern was chosen because HT7 and LU10 are good points for treating the throat. Also, GB39 and ST41 can treat the throat and neck using the

Imaging Format. SI1, SJ1 and LI1 are good for treating stagnation and heat in the head area.

The treatment plan was two treatments per week for three to four weeks, followed by one treatment per week for an additional month. Over the course of treatment, Fatima reported a 75% improvement in her throat discomfort and significantly less neck and back pain. Herbs were also prescribed for the fatigue and depression.

SI1 SJ1 LI1	HT7 LU10 PC8
SP9 KI10 Tan's liver point*	GB39 UB59 ST41

HT7 LU10 PC8	SI1 SJ1 LI1
GB39 UB59 ST41	SP9 KI10 Tan's liver point*

* Located on the medial anterior side of the condyle of the tibia bone. Look for ashi points and use oblique insertion on the bone.

Patterns 3 and 3f

PATTERN 3F

OFFICE MANAGER'S SHOULDER

Thelma, 43, worked for a large home-improvement chain and cared for her invalid mother each day after work. Her chief complaint was shoulder pain from helping her mother in and out of bed. She took pain medication for two years with no improvement in the condition. She was also overweight with a three-year history of mild diabetes, and she suffered from shortness of breath and low energy.

Working on the computer for two to three hours per day aggravated her pain. The range of motion in her entire right

Case Studies

shoulder joint was restricted. Abduction, adduction and extension of her right arm were approximately 50 to 60%. Pattern 3f was chosen to focus on her shoulder while addressing her other complaints. The Shu-Stream and Jing-River points in Group 3 can treat the shoulder using the Reverse Mirroring Format.

HT7 LU10 PC7	SI1 SJ2 LI1
GB39 ST38-ST41 UB57 UB60	SP9A KI10 Tan's liver point*

* Located on the medial anterior side of the condyle of the tibia bone. Look for ashi points and use oblique insertion on the bone.

Pattern 3f

The first two treatments showed no significant pain relief, but extension of the arm was increased to 80%. After three treatments, the shoulder pain reduced significantly and Thelma's energy improved. Lime juice was recommended to help stabilize her blood sugar. Thelma was treated two times per week for six weeks. During this time, the range of motion normalized and her shoulder pain reduced from a pain level 10 to a level 2. She stopped taking pain medication, lost ten pounds and her shortness of breath improved.

PATTERNS 4 AND 4F

THE NOBLE SON

Leo, 40, was a bachelor who took care of his mother for the past 10 years. He would run her errands, take her to the doctor and prepare her meals. Leo suggested hiring a professional

Dr. Tan's Strategy of Twelve Magical Points

caregiver, but his mother felt hurt and abandoned at the idea. Leo also practiced criminal law for a large firm and managed the stress of both situations reasonably well.

He complained of a constant tightness around his sacrum and lower abdomen for about one year. Leo would always wake around 4:00 a.m. to urinate, and he could not fall back asleep. He consistently received less than five hours of sleep each night, and he felt depressed and unmotivated. About six months before seeking treatment, he began to experience burning in the prostate area during urination. His PSA test was normal and his doctor reported no signs of prostate cancer.

Pattern 4 was chosen because the hand Jing-Well points can treat genital problems using the Imaging Format. LI1 is especially effective for men, and SI1 quickly reduces heat and burning sensations.

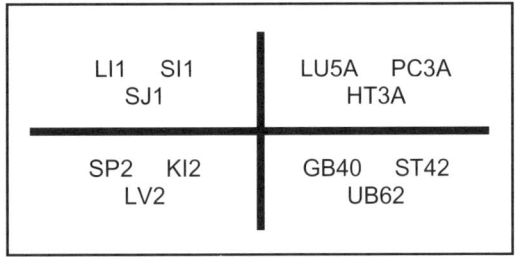

Pattern 4

Leo reported no significant change after the first two treatments. After the third treatment, the burning sensation during urination decreased and he experienced two restful nights of sleep. Pattern 4 was used alternately with 4f. He continued to receive treatments twice per week for six more weeks. The abdominal and sacral tightness disappeared, along with the frequent urination. The burning sensation decreased significantly.

Case Studies

```
LU5A  PC3A    | LI1   SI1
    HT3A      |    SJ1
--------------+--------------
GB40   ST42   | SP2   LV2
    UB62      |    KI2
```

Pattern 4f

Leo continued to have sleep disturbances about every other night. An advanced system of the Balance Method was applied to balance the Jue Yin and Shao Yang meridians. Bilateral Ear Shen Men was also added to the treatment plan. Over the course of ten treatments, the frequency of symptoms was reduced to one night per week. Leo is currently being treated to eliminate his sleeping disorder.

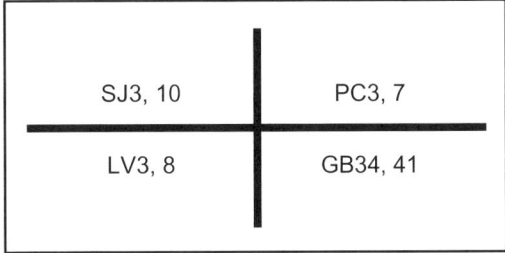

Jue Yin/Shao Yang Combination

PATTERNS 4 AND 4F

THE HIGH PRICE

Gail, 37, was a sales executive for a large electronics firm. Her job demanded travel across the United States each week. She often would eat airplane food and attempt to sleep during the flight. Frequently, she arrived at her destination with a mere

Dr. Tan's Strategy of Twelve Magical Points

four hours of sleep. After about one year, Gail sought treatment for stomach bloating after eating.

Pattern 4 and 4f were chosen due to sensitivity on palpation of the Stomach, Kidney and Gall Bladder channels around her navel. These meridians can be balanced using the arm-yin He-Sea points according to Imaging Format. The two patterns were used alternately during the treatment period. Gail only came for treatments one time per week due to her busy travel schedule. After two treatments, the bloating significantly improved. After one month, she experienced symptoms about once per week when she overate. Herbal medicine was also dispensed to aid in her digestion. Gail received treatments for one more month and was released. She now seeks occasional treatment for stress relief and any flare-ups of the bloating.

LI1 SI1 SJ1	LU5 PC3 HT3	LU5 PC3 HT3	LI1 SI1 SJ1
SP3 KI3 LV3	GB39A ST41 UB59	GB39A ST41 UB59	SP3 KI3 LV3

Patterns 4 and 4f

PATTERNS 4 AND 4F
BEARING THE DUTY

Linda, 46, was a massage therapist who used various styles of energy work on her clients for the past 20 years. Despite working six days per week, Linda appeared relaxed and in good health. However, she sought treatment for an intense feeling of pressure around the neck and shoulders. The discomfort felt like a tight collar around her neck and it had worsened over the

Case Studies

course of two years. It was most severe for about one week before her menses. She also experienced abdominal discomfort around her navel prior to menstrual flow. While her lab tests were normal, Linda felt that menopause was imminent.

Pattern 4 was selected because the Shu-Stream and Jing-River points on the foot are particularly effective for the neck area. She was treated three times per week for three weeks. By the ninth treatment, the intensity of heaviness and tightness decreased from a pain level 10 to level 2. She also experienced a reduction in the abdominal discomfort preceding that month's menstrual period.

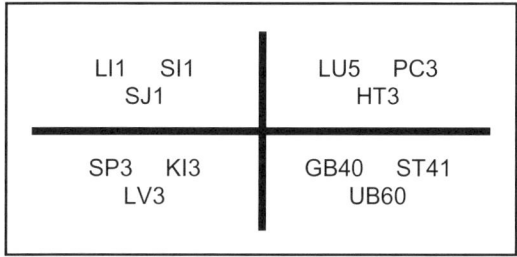

Pattern 4

Patterns 4 and 4f were alternated two times per week for two months. As Linda improved, she only needed two to three treatments during the week before her menses. She maintained this schedule for three menstrual cycles and all of her symptoms disappeared.

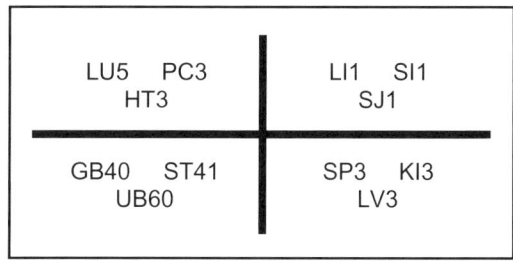

Pattern 4f

PATTERN 5

MICKEY'S "MOUSE" SYNDROME

Mickey, 45, spent most of his time on the computer. He enjoyed exploring the internet and consequently developed "mouse" syndrome from repetitive use of the computer mouse. Mickey felt right-sided elbow pain after about five hours on the computer.

Mickey also had left-sided headaches around his temples and behind his eyes. These headaches were often accompanied by insomnia. He also suffered from nausea and left-sided discomfort in his rib area.

The first treatment plan began with Systems 1 and 3 of the Balance Method. GB31, 32, 33 and 34A were used on the left side to treat Shao Yang elbow pain. LV3 was needled on the right side to treat the headache. After five treatments using this protocol, Mickey's headaches and rib tightness improved and the elbow pain decreased. However, there was still elbow pain in the areas around SI8 and LI11, and Mickey still suffered with nausea. Pattern 5 was selected after the fifth treatment. After one treatment with this pattern, all the symptoms were relieved.

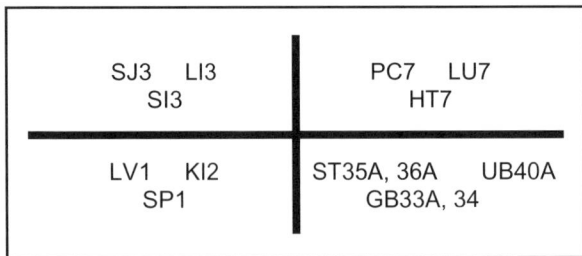

Pattern 5

Case Studies

PATTERN 5

AFFLICTIONS FOR ALCHEMY

Marla was a 30-year-old computer software engineer. Her job was very stressful and she only remained in the position due to the slow job market. She developed pain in her right shoulder from overuse on the computer. The discomfort often extended into the right scapula and neck. She rated the pain at a constant level of 4-5, but the severity increased to a level 7-9 with daily use. In addition, Marla suffered with menstrual cramps, premenstrual moodiness, headaches, occasional insomnia and digestive problems. She commented on her feelings of unworthiness and added stress from romantic relationships. Marla felt overwhelmed and wondered if acupuncture could treat all her symptoms. She joked that only magic could help all her problems.

The pain in the upper shoulder included the areas around SI12, GB20, GB21 and LI16. Pattern 5 was selected to address the chief complaint. The yin Shu-Stream and Jing-River points can effectively treat the neck and shoulder pain according to the Systems of the Balance Method.

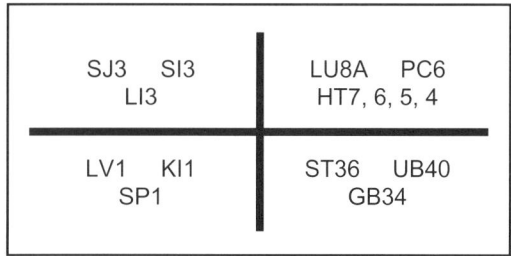

Pattern 5

Marla returned two days later and was very satisfied with her first treatment. She no longer had constant discomfort, and the pain was reduced to 50% even after working continuously on the computer. She also had more energy, two restful nights of sleep and no digestive disturbance.

She received three treatments per week for three weeks. Her pain decreased 90% since her first visit. Marla was also given herbal medicine after the first two treatments for her menstrual problems and sleep imbalances. She had no P.M.S. symptoms with her next menstrual cycle. Her treatments were then reduced to two times per week for three more weeks, and then reduced to one time per week for one month.

PATTERNS 5 AND 5F
MILLER'S SADNESS

Miller, 50, was a tough woman who owned a successful business. She survived breast cancer after a radical mastectomy on the right side, but she had lingering pain in the area of the surgery. Her illness and pain left her angry and depressed. She often experienced insomnia, low energy and intermittent headaches. She requested that no needles be inserted in her right upper arm due to the removal of the lymph glands in this region.

Patterns 5 and 5f were used alternately, and the right upper limb points were not needled.

	PC7 LU7 HT7		SJ3 SI3 LI3
LV1 KI1 SP1	ST36 UB40 GB34	ST36 UB40 GB34	LV1 KI1 SP1

Patterns 5 and 5f

Case Studies

After four treatments, Miller experienced more energy, restful sleep and a 50% decrease in her pain. She continued treatments three times per week for three more weeks. All her symptoms were controlled, including the depression. Miller travels frequently for business and now comes for maintenance treatments every one to two months.

PATTERN 6
THE HANDS OF THE MASTER BUILDER

Glenn was a 41-year-old carpenter who learned his trade from his father since he was a young boy. Constructing beautiful homes had been his whole life. Over the years, both of his hands began to ache from constant use. His right palm was most painful, and he felt tingling in the second, fourth and fifth fingertips on the right hand.

Glenn also experienced dizziness on a daily basis. After running considerable medical tests, his doctor told Glenn that he may have an inner ear problem. Pattern 6 was selected in order to address the chief complaint on the hands. The Jing-Well and Shu-Stream points on the feet most effectively treat the fingertips and the palm when applying the Mirroring concept.

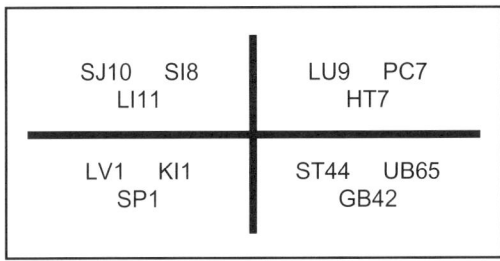

Pattern 6

After the first treatment, Glenn reported less dizziness and a reduction in low back pain. His low back problem was not mentioned during the initial visit. The frequency of the hand tingling was reduced, but the intensity of pain remained unchanged. Glenn continued to work during the course of treatment, and therefore it took more time to stabilize his condition. He received twenty treatments over the course of ten weeks. Over this period, his pain and tingling decreased by 70%.

He continued to receive bi-weekly treatments for another ten weeks. His dizziness was resolved and his back pain disappeared. Glenn still has 10-20% of the initial pain that flares up with overuse. He seeks treatment during these episodes, and the Mirroring Format of the Balance Method is applied to focus on his hands.

PATTERN 6F

THE SINGER'S MALADY

Kate, 68, was a jazz singer who performed her whole life. As a small child, she would sing in church every week. She recalled the intense stage fright before each performance. On Sunday mornings, her nervousness manifested as diarrhea and neck pain. She conquered the performance anxiety over the years, yet her throat always felt constricted despite relaxation exercises for her neck muscles. She complained of a tightness in the front portion of her neck and throat irritation when swallowing. She caught frequent colds that lingered in her throat and rarely moved deeper into the lungs. Kate also experienced Irritable Bowel Syndrome with alternating constipation and loose stools for more than ten years.

Case Studies

Pattern 6f was selected because Group 3 can address the neck and throat areas when using the Imaging Format. Also, LI11 images the abdominal area and therefore treats bowel disorders.

PC7 HT7 LU9, 10	LI11, 10 SJ10 S18
GB43 ST44 UB65	LV1 SP1 KI2

Pattern 6f

Kate felt no significant change after the first three treatments. After the fourth treatment, her neck tightness significantly diminished and she was having two firm bowel movements everyday. She received treatments two times per week for six weeks and her irritable bowel disorder completely resolved. However, Kate still had the urge to swallow often due to a blocked sensation in her throat similar to plum-pit qi stagnation. Pattern 6f was revised to image the throat area in all four-segments. After one more month, Kate was released with no throat or symptoms.

PC7 HT7 LU9, 10	LI5 SJ4 SI5
GB40 ST41 UB62	LV2 SP2 KI6

Pattern 6f Revised

Dr. Tan's Strategy of Twelve Magical Points

PATTERN 6

NUMBER PAIN

Debbie, 39, worked on data entry in an accounting department. She had suffered from right-sided migraine headaches for 15 years. She described the pain as a cold sensation, along with tightness in her neck. Her headaches worsened in frequency and intensity despite prescription medications. She also experienced spasmodic flank pain along the Gall Bladder channel on her right side. These conditions often occurred simultaneously and intensified her pain.

Pattern 6 was chosen because HT4 is extremely effective for neck pain, and the San Jiao points can treat the flank pain. All twelve of the Magic Points relieve headache pain. After the first treatment, Debbie only experienced one headache in four days. She took Ibuprofen and the headache lasted only two hours. Pattern 6 was applied two times per week for five weeks. The frequency of the headaches decreased from every day to twice per week. The intensity of pain decreased from level 10 to level 2, and she stopped taking pain medications. Her flank pain also improved by 80%. Due to financial concerns, treatments were reduced to once a week. After two months, Debbie was released without any pain.

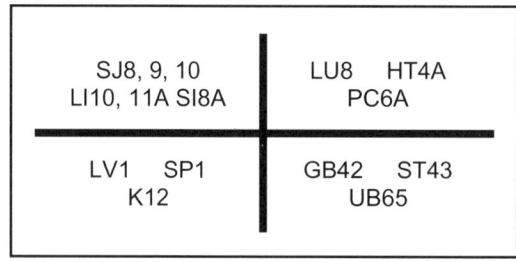

Pattern 6

Case Studies

PATTERNS 7 AND 7F
CLEAR AS A BREATH

Susan was a 22-year-old college student who suffered from severe allergies to pollen and dust since she was a small child. Her sinuses became blocked with white and clear mucus, and she experienced profuse post-nasal drip. She suffered with sinus headaches above her eyebrows and temples, and the pain would encompass her whole head.

Patterns 7 and 7f were chosen because the hands can treat the head and throat under the Imaging Format. During the first treatment, Susan's nasal area opened and her breathing cleared. The recommended treatment plan was three treatments per week for four to five weeks. The instantaneous results convinced her to move forward with the treatments.

LU10 PC8 HT8	LI4 SI5 SJ4		LI4 SI5 SJ4	LU10 PC8 HT8
GB44 ST45 UB67	SP9 KI10 LV8		SP9 KI10 LV8	GB44 ST45 UB67

Patterns 7 and 7f

Susan's symptoms were 50% better after five treatments. Herbal medicine was prescribed in conjunction with her acupuncture treatments. By the end of the fifth week, all of her symptoms were significantly reduced. During periods of high pollen count, she experienced some sneezing in the morning but remained headache free. Susan was released after nine treatments and occasionally returns for aggravations of her symptoms.

PATTERN 7F
THE FLOOR MANAGER'S FOOT

Mark was a 43-year-old warehouse manager for a heating and ventilation company. Due to layoffs, his work included manual labor, extensive paperwork and the supervision of an understaffed shipping department. Mark suffered from left-sided foot pain in the tarsal bones. He experienced aching and burning along the dorsal part of the foot and ankle, from the medial to the lateral side. He did not recall any specific injury, and there was no discoloration or swelling.

The initial treatment stage began with the Balance Method. The right hand was needled between the carpal bones to mirror the affected area on the left foot. The patient's condition stabilized after five treatments.

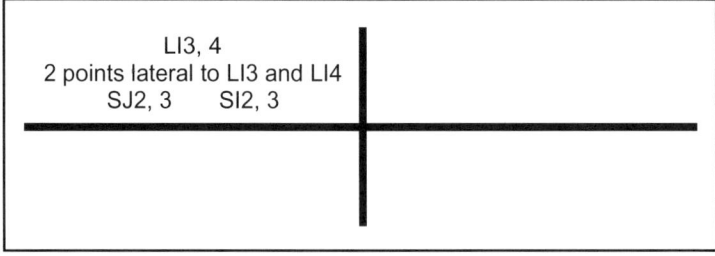

Mirroring Format

At this time, Mark wondered if acupuncture could help his other complaints. He suffered from abdominal pain accompanied by a headache one day per week. Medical treatments proved ineffective and showed no pathology. Pattern 7f was selected because Group 3 could still effectively treat his foot pain while his other complaints were addressed. After the first treatment, the headache and abdominal discomfort significantly decreased. Mark was treated twice per week for three more weeks and his

Case Studies

symptoms disappeared. Four more treatments were administered to stabilize the condition and he was advised to seek treatments if any symptoms recurred. Mark has not returned for more than one year.

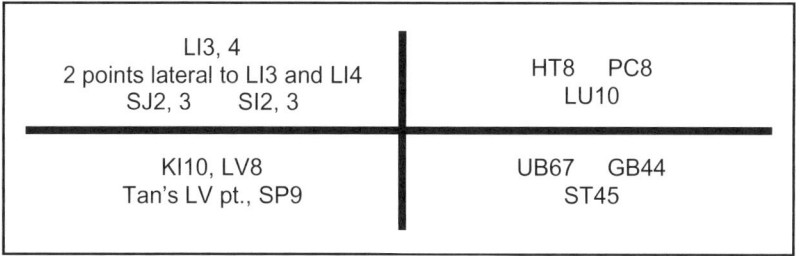

Pattern 7f

PATTERNS 7 AND 7F

ALICE'S PLACEBO

Alice was a 51-year-old elementary school teacher whose job became increasingly stressful over the past ten years. She had been diagnosed with fibromyalgia and chronic fatigue syndrome, however she did not report significant body aches or muscle pain. Alice suffered from daily headaches around her eyes, nose and jaw. She woke up with a sore throat every morning which diminished throughout the day until she became tired. Then, the sore throat would return and remain for the rest of the day. Alice became more and more depressed, and western medications did not help her symptoms.

Pattern 7 and 7f were selected because the upper body points can treat the throat by applying the Imaging Format. The two strategies were alternated with each treatment.

Dr. Tan's Strategy of Twelve Magical Points

LU10 PC7	LI5 SI5	LI5 SI5	LU10 PC7
HT8	SJ4	SJ4	HT7
GB44 ST45	SP9 KI10	SP9 KI10	GB44 ST45
UB67	LV8	LV8	UB67

Patterns 7 and 7f

After three treatments, Alice experienced a 10-15% decrease in the intensity and frequency of her symptoms. Alice wondered if this was a placebo effect, yet she continued treatments. Ten treatments later, Alice only had minimal headache pain. She still experienced sore throats on a daily basis, but the pain had lessened. She received treatments two times per week for seven weeks. The headaches completely disappeared and her sore throats now occurred every 3-4 days. She experienced more energy, better sleep and her depression lifted. Alice was released with no symptoms after eight additional treatments.

PATTERN 8

MONTHLY ENDURANCE

Lois, 34, was a banking executive who exercised each morning at 4:30 a.m. and did not return home from work until about 7:30pm. For several years, Lois had suffered with severe cramps that began one day before her menstrual flow and continued for two days during her menses. Her physician prescribed birth control pills which gave her little relief. In addition to the cramps, she experienced sharp headaches behind her eyes. She also complained of tingling in her left fingers upon waking during the night or in the morning.

Case Studies

Pattern 8 was selected because the Jing-Well points on the right foot effectively treat the left fingers. The initial treatment plan was one treatment per week, along with three treatments during the week prior to menses.

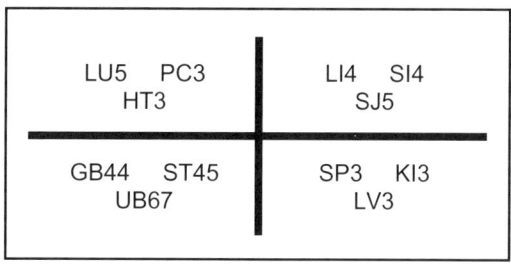

Pattern 8

After six treatments, her cramping and headache pain decreased from a pain level 10 to level 4 during her next menstrual cycle. The treatment plan continued for three menstrual cycles and the pain was reduced to level 1. Lois then received treatments only during the week before her menses. Following four menstrual cycles, Lois no longer experienced headaches, cramps or tingling in her fingers.

PATTERNS 8 AND 8F
THE JOY OF REPOSE

Joy, 52, was a teacher and art historian. She was a sensitive woman who became easily upset and was somewhat obsessive in her work. She experienced heart palpitations before falling asleep each night, and she sometimes felt her heart skip a beat. She slept well during the night, yet she woke up with a dry mouth and bitter taste. Her pulse felt bouncy but showed no irregularity in the beat.

Dr. Tan's Strategy of Twelve Magical Points

Pattern 1 was selected first because the yin Jing-Well points on the hands are most effective in treating palpitations.

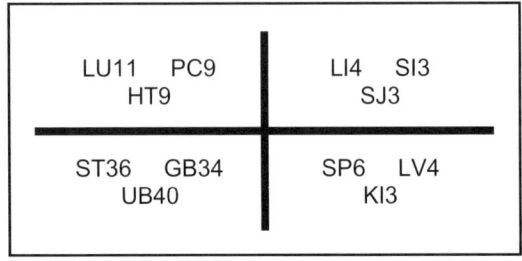

Pattern 1

Joy was a piano player and despised the needling of the Jing-Well points on her hand. Therefore, the treatment strategy was adjusted to Patterns 8 and 8f. The two strategies were administered alternately with each treatment.

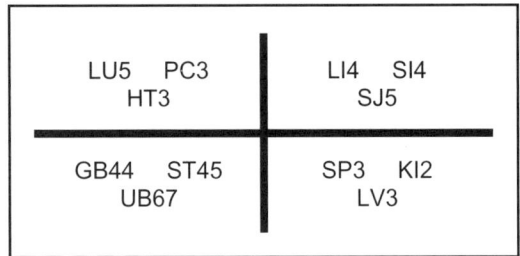

Pattern 8

After the first six treatments, Joy reported a lessening in her the palpitations. She was unsure if the acupuncture helped her condition because a nutritional consultant advised a change in her vitamin regimen. She decided to stop taking all of her supplements during the next course of acupuncture treatments. After three treatments per week for three weeks, she experienced only one incident of palpitations every five days.

Case Studies

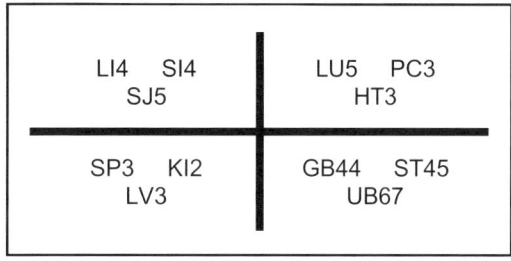

Pattern 8f

The treatments were reduced to two times per week for four more weeks. Joy responded with more energy and her palpitations disappeared.

PATTERN 8
RUNNING RELIEF

Jess was a 38-year-old salesman for a printing company. After his wife was laid off from her job, he experienced emotional stress from the financial difficulties and resulting domestic turmoil. Jess typically played tennis and jogged several times a week to relieve stress and stay healthy. For six months, Jess experienced pain in his right lateral malleolus at the end of each day. He also complained of lower leg pain and tightness in a four-inch area from his femur to the knee.

Jess also felt a decrease in his energy for about one year, and he occasionally experienced episodes of dizziness and blurred vision after eating lunch. All medical tests were normal.

Pattern 8 was chosen because the upper Shu-Stream and Jing-River points on the left side can effectively address right-sided ankle and leg pain. In addition, the upper yin He-Sea points treat vision problems using the Imaging Format.

Dr. Tan's Strategy of Twelve Magical Points

```
┌─────────────────────┬─────────────────────┐
│   LU5    PC3        │   LI5-6    SI5-7    │
│      HT3            │      SJ4, 5         │
├─────────────────────┼─────────────────────┤
│   GB44   ST45       │    SP3    KI2       │
│      UB67           │       LV3           │
└─────────────────────┴─────────────────────┘
```

Pattern 8

The treatment plan consisted of three treatments per week. After two weeks, his ankle pain decreased by 75%. The dizziness was reduced and his blurred vision improved significantly. Jess still felt some tightness around the lateral malleolus after running or playing tennis. The treatment plan was adjusted to two treatments per week for four more weeks. After one month, Jess was released symptom free. He occasionally receives treatments for stress relief.

Appendix A: Pattern Comparison by Sequential Direction of Groups

Dr. Tan's Strategy of Twelve Magical Points

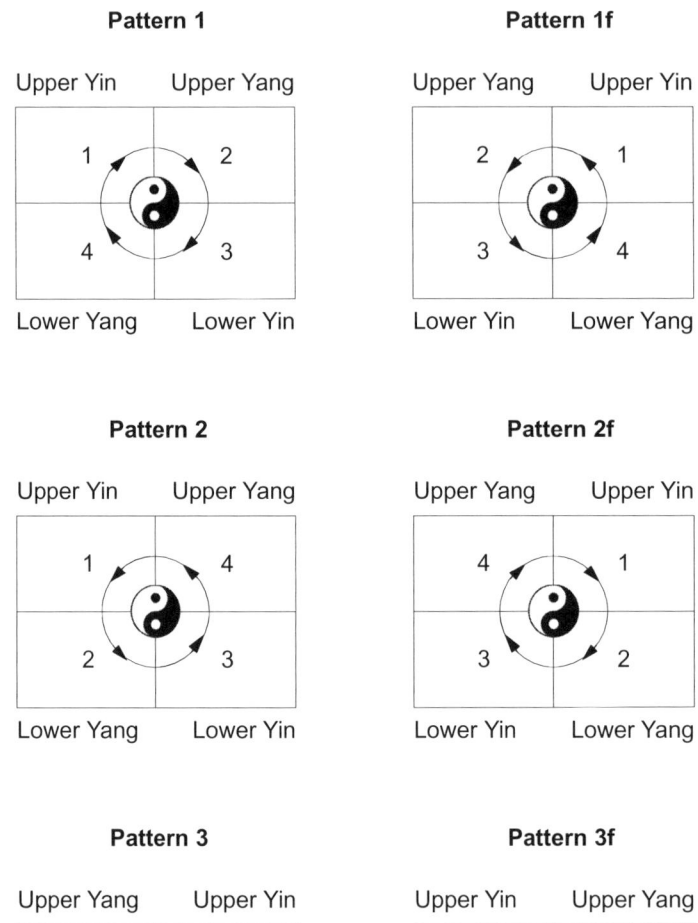

Appendix A: Pattern Comparison by Sequential Direction of

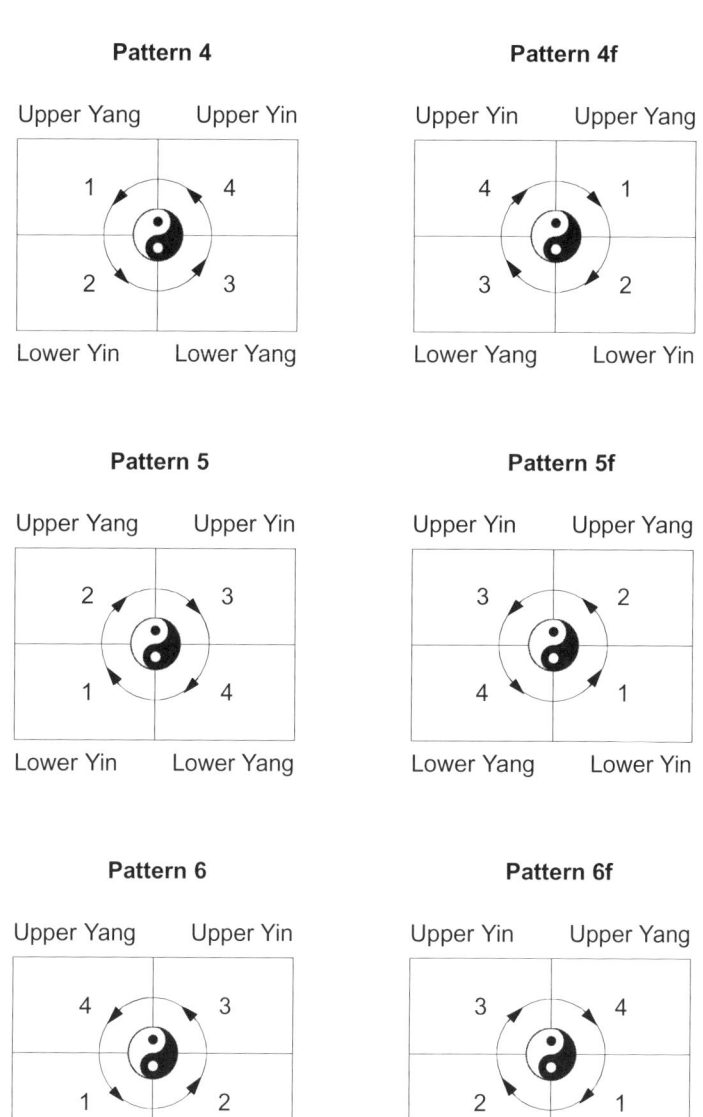

Dr. Tan's Strategy of Twelve Magical Points

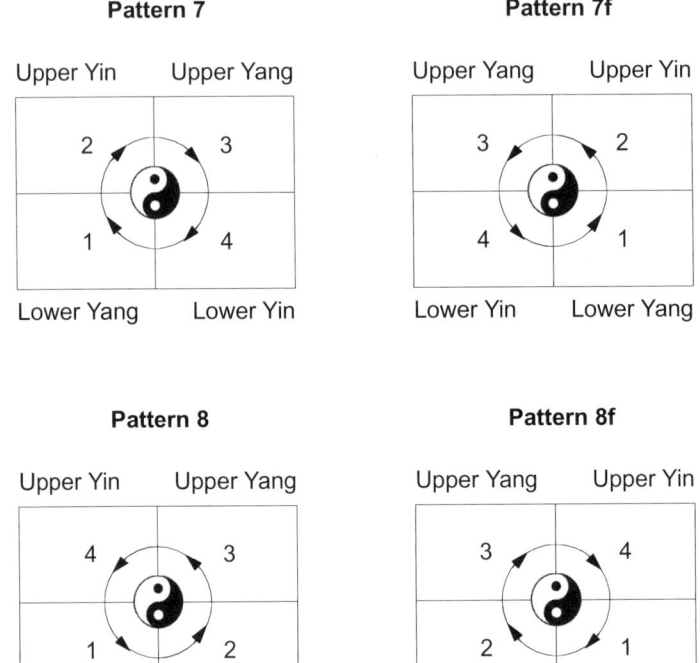

Appendix B: Commonly Asked Questions

Can I use local points from my current style of acupuncture treatment with distal points of the Balance Method?

It is not suggested to combine different styles of treatment with the Balance Method. The focus of the chosen system is dissipated and generally will not deliver efficient results.

Is exact textbook location of a point necessary for good results?

The "ashi", or most sensitive area around the point, is recommended for the best response to the treatment. Exact point location is not as essential as finding ashi points in the chosen area.

Dr. Tan's Strategy of Twelve Magical Points

My patients are not accustomed to strong stimulation of the needles. Is this necessary to achieve good results from the Balance Method?

Chi sensation is required for clinical results. However, the strength of needle stimulation may need to be adjusted based on individual patient sensitivity. Some patients feel a strong sensation with minimal stimulation, while other patients are less sensitive to the needles.

How long should I retain the needles?

The needles should be retained 45-60 minutes, as it often takes 10-15 minutes for the patient to reach a relaxed state.

How frequent should I see my patients for maximum results?

Daily treatment may be necessary for severe pain that returns quickly between treatments. In general, patients should be treated before the pain is allowed to reach its original level. This usually requires 2-3 treatments per week in the initial treatment stages.

Many of my patients insist on continuing to exercise during the treatment period. Can this effect the outcome of the treatments?

Any activity that aggravates the pain or discomfort should be eliminated until the condition improves. Progress of the condition will take much longer if the patient continues to re-injure the area.

Other Books by Richard Tan

In-depth information about Dr. Tan's books and seminars can be found on the web at: *http://www.drtanshow.com*.

Twelve and Twelve in Acupuncture

The first in a series of books by Richard Tan, L.Ac., O.M.D. and Stephen Rush, L.Ac. focusing on unique acupuncture point usage and case studies for the dramatic and highly effective method of pain treatment by use of distal point strategy. See the order form on the following pages.

Twenty Four More in Acupuncture

The second in a series of books by Richard Tan, L.Ac., O.M.D. and Stephen Rush, L.Ac. focusing on unique acupuncture point usage and case studies for the dramatic and highly effective method of pain treatment by use of distal point strategy. This book is a "must have" for those who have the first book in the series, *Twelve and Twelve in Acupuncture*. See the order form on the following pages.

Dr. Tan's Strategy of Twelve Magical Points

Shower of Jewels
FENG SHUI: AN AMUSING YET PRACTICAL GUIDE TO ANCIENT PRINCIPLES OF PLACEMENT AND GEOENERGY MANIPULATION

By Richard Tan, L.Ac., O.M.D. and Cheryl Warnke, L.Ac. Shower of Jewels is the most easy-to-understand and applicable book on the market about Feng Shui to date. No longer do you or your patients need to feel like hapless victims of their surroundings and circumstances. By using Feng Shui principles you can gain the power to create an environment to work to your advantage. See the order form on the following pages.

To order ***Twelve and Twelve in Acupuncture*** or ***Twenty-Four More in Acupuncture***:
Check or credit card: $30.00 per book (includes $5.00 shipping and handling)

To order ***Shower of Jewels***:
Check or credit card: $31.00 per book (includes $5.00 shipping and handling)

To order ***Dr. Tan's Strategy of Twelve Magical Points***:
Check or credit card: $29.00 per book (includes $5.00 shipping and handling)

Order Form:

Name

Address

City, State, Zip

Phone

Book title(s)
1. _____
2. _____
3. _____
4. _____

Total payment $ _____

Checks payable to: Richard Tan

Credit card: ☐ Visa ☐ MasterCard Exp. Date: _____

Signature _____

Mail order form and payment to:
Richard Tan
4550 Kearny Villa Rd., #107
San Diego, CA 92123

Fax order form to:
(858) 277-9037

Book orders may also be placed online at: www.drtranshow.com

Dr. Tan's Strategy of Twelve Magical Points